# TETANUS

# TETANUS

E. B. ADAMS

B.Sc.(Oxon.), M.D.(Rand), F.R.C.P.(Lond.)

*Professor of Medicine*
*University of Natal, Durban*

D. R. LAURENCE

M.D., F.R.C.P.(Lond.)

*Professor of Pharmacology*
*and Therapeutics,*
*University College and*
*University College Hospital*
*Medical School, London*

J. W. G. SMITH

M.D.(Wales), M.C.Path.,
Dip.Bact.(Lond.)

*Head of Bacteriology,*
*Wellcome Research Laboratories,*
*Beckenham, Kent*

Blackwell Scientific Publications
Oxford and Edinburgh

SBN 632 06090 5

First Published 1969

*Printed in Great Britain by*
BILLING AND SONS LTD, GUILDFORD
*and bound by*
THE KEMP HALL BINDERY, OXFORD

# CONTENTS

# PREFACE

This book is written primarily for those who are concerned with tetanus prevention and treatment. In addition to practical aspects we have tried to give in outline the experimental and laboratory background to clinical practice. Each of us has been actively engaged in investigating some of the problems related to tetanus and we have tried to relate our experience to the work of others so as to produce a balanced account of this disease which involves so many disciplines.

In 1940 Dietrich wrote, 'a complete résumé of the literature on the treatment of tetanus would be monumental, confusing, definitely contradictory and of little aid to the physician attempting to treat a single child with tetanus. I shall not attempt it.' We feel the same applies to all aspects of tetanus, whether epidemiology, pharmacology, immunology, bacteriology or treatment. We have therefore been selective, particularly with the references, and we can only hope that any contributor to the field who sees this book and who feels his work has not had the attention it deserves will forgive us. In addition, some of the more detailed and controversial experimental work with no present bearing on clinical practice has been omitted or referred to in passing, although indications of where it may be found have generally been given.

A substantial amount of the clinical research with which the authors have been concerned has been generously supported by the Wellcome Trust. It is a pleasure to thank the Trustees.

We are also indebted to many colleagues, without whose assistance much of this work would not have been possible. In particular we thank Drs M. K. Sykes, N. M. Mann, R. Holloway, A. K. Thambiran, Anne Wesley, S. D. Desai, B. G. Jackson and R. Wright, as well as the sisters, nurses and technical staff of the Respiratory Unit, King Edward VIII Hospital, Durban. We also acknowledge the co-operation and facilities provided by the Natal Provincial Administration.

Prof. A. J. Wilmot kindly read and commented on the manuscript, and Mrs J. R. Rudder was responsible for its typing and careful checking; we are grateful to both for their help.

E. B. Adams
D. R. Laurence
J. W. G. Smith

# I

# HISTORICAL INTRODUCTION

Clear descriptions of tetanus occur in the literature throughout medical history, for the typical severe case is easily recognized and runs a short course, often ending in death. Hippocrates wrote that victims 'die within four days, or if they pass these they recover'.

In time when most, or indeed the only, accurate part of medical texts was the description of the patient seen from the bedside, various terms were coined to describe the postures resulting from local variations in the intensity of muscle contraction—opisthotonos, orthotonos, pleurosthotonos and emprosthotonos, but except for the first, they are now obsolete. One possible reason is that the physician is no longer compelled to stand by for days observing the unchecked manifestations of the disease, and another that they carry no particular diagnostic or prognostic value.

Until the introduction of volatile general anaesthetics in the middle of the 19th century, the physician relied chiefly on opium and a variety of strange and futile methods in his attempts to arrest the disease. He lacked both the knowledge and the means for effective therapy. The treatments he used make an interesting catologue: amputation, hot baths, cold baths, blisters, eserine, digitalis, tobacco, hydrocyanic acid, quinine, aconite, mercury, ipecacuanha, amyl nitrite, acupuncture, and, inevitably, bleeding by leeches or by venesection.

The first hint of a rational therapeutic approach came when the muscle-paralysing effect of crude curare preparations from South America became known to medicine. In 1811, Benjamin Brodie showed that artificial respiration with a bellows (intermittent positive pressure respiration) preserved the life of curarized animals and suggested that it might be useful in tetanus. This disease was indeed the subject of the first attempt to use curare in therapeutics, in animals in 1835, and in man in 1858, when the crude preparation was applied to the wound. In 1859, Spencer Wells injected it in three cases. He reported that after one injection of a crude preparation the patient 'fell backwards as if dead, and the pulse and respiration both stopped for several seconds . . . I was unable to satisfy myself whether this faintness was a mere effect of the puncture, of which she had expressed dread, or of the action of the woorara. . . . If the latter (perhaps) I had accidentally punctured a small vein and thrown the solution directly into the circulation.'

His account also illustrates the existing ignorance about the pathogenesis of post-operative tetanus. The disease had occurred in three of his gynaecological cases in 4 weeks and he ascribed it to a cold draught in the ward and to surgical injury to the nerves. He mentioned the possibility that the wound might develop a 'perverted secretion' but did not consider the likelihood of a common source of infection; the nature of the disease was to remain obscure for a further 25 years. Wells suggested 'very respectfully' to the fellows of the Royal Medical and Chirurgical Society of London that 'more accurate observation of what may be called the Natural History of Tetanus is much needed'.

At this time climate was widely thought to be important, and case reports sometimes included meteorological data: 'tetanus set in twenty-eight days after the injury on July 5th, 1825. Cloudy and hazy, north winds, W., N.E., N.; temperature 65° to 70°' (Poland 1857).

Few were able to take as detached a view as Cullen (1827) who, stating his ignorance of the pathology, added that 'in such a situation, therefore, the endeavouring to give any rules of practice, upon a scientific plan, appears to me vain and fruitless'. He employed large doses of opium, but recommended 'the frequent exhibition of laxatives while the power of deglutition remains, or the frequent exhibition of clysters where it does not: and the good effects of both have been frequently observed'.

The initial failure of curare in therapeutics was inevitable because the crude preparations could not be standardized and so accurate dosage was impossible. In addition, even if a reliable preparation had been available, its use would have foundered in the absence of efficient means of long-term artificial respiration since it is not possible to control tetanus convulsions adequately by neuromuscular block without abolishing spontaneous respiration. For these reasons the use of curare and intermittent positive pressure respiration as a serious therapeutic enterprise had to wait until the middle of the present century, when the necessary technical skills were developed.

Meanwhile, central nervous system depressants of all kinds have been used in tetanus. Some of them, such as paraldehyde, chloral, barbiturates, mephenesin, chlorpromazine and diazepam, are widely used and remain the basis of therapy in many parts of the world. The qualities desired of an anticonvulsant in tetanus are that it should control reflex convulsions so that they occur infrequently, are brief, and do not arrest respiration; so far the ideal has not been found.

Antitoxin was introduced into prophylaxis (p. 45) and therapy in about 1897, but only recently has convincing clinical evidence been added to the presumption that it should be beneficial after the disease has developed. This delay may seem strange, but it is really what is to be expected. Toxin 'fixed' (p. 107) to the central nervous system is not neutralizable, so any benefit which may result from the therapeutic use of antitoxin will depend on the extent to which neutralization of unfixed toxin reduces the ultimate severity of the disease. Moreover, patients with tetanus die of a wide variety of complications only partially related to the amount of toxin free at the time of diagnosis, when antitoxin is given.

Comparative evaluation of therapy to the standards of the modern controlled therapeutic trial has been attempted only recently in tetanus, and in some aspects of the disease nothing has been done. There are many reasons for this, including the fact that large numbers of cases are liable to be needed because of the multiple causes of death. For instance, elimination of one factor such as *Cl. tetani* from the wound, which is presumptively desirable, would be unlikely to be followed by any detectable effect on the fatality rate in any series of reasonable size; prevention of respiratory infection, if successful, might only show an effect in a large series, and so on. Other reasons are that tetanus is common where medical services are least developed, the controlled therapeutic trial has, until recent years been almost confined to areas where the disease is relatively rare, and such trials have been thought impracticable in tetanus.

The literature of tetanus consists largely of reports of single cases in which survival was thought to be worth recording because of the treatment used; surveys of series of cases, often large, in which the unsually low mortality was attributed to whatever therapeutic innovation the authors happen to have made recently; and short series of consecutive recoveries, published with similar claims.

Creech, Glover and Ochsner (1957), reviewing the experience at the Charity Hospital, New Orleans (U.S.A.), stated that lack of understanding of the pathogenesis of tetanus, together with uncontrolled variables which alter the course of the disease, make it difficult if not impossible to assess the effectiveness of various forms of therapy. They particularly condemned conclusions drawn from small series. In one series of 15 consecutive recoveries which they cite, the authors concluded that central depressant drugs were highly effective. Creech and his colleagues pointed out that in 1949 'there were 52 cases of tetanus observed at the Charity Hospital and of these, 19 consecutive patients survived. Yet, the mortality for that year was 42 per cent. It is apparent that the treatment employed in the 19 consecutive survivors might have been credited with the successful outcome. The fact is, however, that cases prior to and subsequent to these 19 were treated essentially in the same fashion with singularly poor results.'

The modern controlled therapeutic trial as defined by Bradford Hill is 'a carefully and ethically designed experiment with the aim of answering some precisely framed question. In its most rigorous form it demands equivalent groups of patients concurrently treated in different ways. These groups are constructed by the random allocation of patients to one or other treatment. . . . In principle the method is applicable with any disease and any treatment. It may also be applied on any scale; it does not necessarily demand large numbers of patients.' The controlled trial can be carried out in tetanus—there are examples in this book—and should be done more often. It provides the only reliable way of identifying improvements in therapy that fall short of the dramatic and of avoiding false conclusions from the impressions of uncontrolled experience.

It is nevertheless important to avoid unthinking reliance on these techniques. Where the natural history of a disease is reliably predictable, as in tuberculous meningitis and tetanus neonatorum, a substantial improvement in results may be attributed to treatment even in the absence of carefully controlled studies. For example, if in a large series of infants with tetanus neonatorum only 20 per cent die, it would be irrational to ignore this striking improvement because the study was uncontrolled, since the case fatality rate is ordinarily above 80 per cent. If, however, in such a series 70 per cent had died, it would be impossible to attribute this slight improvement to any given treatment. Enormous advances in treatment are detectable without controlled studies, but unfortunately enormous advances are rare and cannot be predicted. The controlled study therefore offers the most ethical and the most economical and surest way to advance knowledge.

Because tetanus has been such a prominent feature of major wars until that of 1939–45, when it presented no problem, it is interesting to look briefly at this aspect of history. Boyd (1958) divides wars and campaigns into three categories for the incidence of tetanus in the wounded:

| | cases per 1000 wounded |
|---|---|
| 1 *Before specific prophylaxis of any kind* | |
| British forces in Spain (Peninsular War), 1808–14 | 12·5 |
| Crimean War, 1854–56 | 2·0 |
| American Civil War, 1861–65 | 2·0 |
| Franco-Prussian War, 1870–71 | 3·5 |
| 2 *Where passive immunization alone was available* | |
| Western Front, 1914–18 | 1·47 |
| 3 *Where both active and passive immunization were available* | |
| British Expeditionary Force, 1939–40 | 0·43 |
| North-West Europe, 1944–45 | 0·06 |
| United States Army, 1942–45 | 0·0062 |

The true picture for the British Army is better than the figures suggest, for all the cases in the Expeditionary Force 1939–40 are known to have been in soldiers who 'dodged' inoculation with toxoid, and so are half of those in 1944–45. The figure for the United States Army represents a single case out of 160,254 wounded (there were 11 other cases of tetanus in the U.S. Army but they were not due to battle wounds).

Despite the fact that the type of ground over which the campaigns were fought, the availability of surgery and other factors must have had considerable influence, it remains reasonable to attribute much of the decline of tetanus in war to the effective provision of immunological prophylaxis.

# 2

# BACTERIOLOGY

The genus *Clostridium*, to which the causative organism of tetanus belongs, contains those Gram-positive bacilli that grow only under anaerobic conditions and which are able for form endospores. The group includes a number of species that produce powerful toxins and are dangerous pathogens for man and animals, e.g. the causative organism of botulism, *Clostridium botulinum*, and the gas-gangrene organisms—*Cl. welchii* (or *Cl. perfringens* as it may also be called), *Cl. oedematiens* (or *Cl. novyi*) and *Cl. septicum*. The genus also includes a variety of species which are non-pathogenic saprophytes, e.g. *Cl. sporogenes*, *Cl. tetanomorphum*. The individual species of the spore-bearing anaerobes are identified in the laboratory by means of their biochemical activities, in particular their ability to break down proteins and carbohydrates, and in the case of the pathogenic species, by means of their toxins which are often the major factors determining the pathogenicity of the clostridia. Thus the ability of *Cl. tetani* to cause human disease is attributable, perhaps entirely, to the powerful neurotoxin it produces, and pathogenic strains can readily be recognized in the laboratory by demonstrating that they produce this toxin.

## *Habitat*

*Cl. tetani* is commonly to be found in soil and in the faeces of domestic animals and, not infrequently, in human faeces. It seems likely that the main natural habitat of tetanus bacilli is the soil, but isolation is most frequently successful when the earth samples are taken from cultivated ground rich in animal manure. It has been demonstrated that multiplication of the bacilli can occur in rich soil (see Bytchenko 1966), but there is also evidence that they can multiply in the large intestine of guinea-pigs (Tenbroeck & Bauer 1924), although it is not known if multiplication occurs in the intestine of carnivores or of man. The possibility thus remains that the continued presence of the bacilli in soil is dependent on the deposition of faecal material.

From soil and faeces *Cl. tetani* contaminates the human environment; spores can be recovered from house dust, clothing and also from the air of occupied places, including hospitals (see p. 35) (Lowbury & Lilly 1958).

## *Morphology*

The organisms found in an overnight growth of most strains of *Cl. tetani* are actively motile bacilli about $5\text{–}8 \times 0{\cdot}4\mu$ in size, although filamentous forms of up to about $30\mu$ are not uncommonly seen in swarming cultures on solid media. The characteristic drum-stick appearance of the spore-bearing bacilli may be seen but, since sporulation is influenced by various factors such as the age of the culture, the nature of the growth medium, and the particular strain being studied, spores may be absent.

*Cl. tetani* is typically Gram-positive but, like many clostridia, in older cultures the organisms may become Gram-variable or frankly Gram-negative; indeed this may be the case in cultures only 24 hours' old. In old cultures the spherical spores only may be present, and these are seen indistinctly in Gram-stained films.

The spore-bearing bacillus does not invariably show the typical drum-stick appearance and in some strains the spore is distinctly oval and subterminal. Indeed, the immature spore often appears oval in shape, and the mature spore may also appear slightly oval, owing to the presence of what appears to be a fragment of the original bacterial cytoplasm remaining adherent to the spore. Spores may develop at each end of a bacillus giving a 'dumb-bell' appearance. The drum-stick appearance is not confined to *Cl. tetani*—it is seen in the saprophyte *Cl. tetanomorphum*, as its name implies.

## *Cultural characteristics*

*Cl. tetani* is a strict anaerobe, and it has been shown that spores require an oxidation-reduction potential (Eh) of $+0{\cdot}01$ volts or less at *p*H 7·0 in order to germinate (Fildes 1929). The optimum growth temperature is about 37°C, but growth occurs, although very slowly, at 22°C. It grows well on the usual rich laboratory media such as digest agar and blood agar, with the production of a faintly rancid odour. Maximum growth may not be evident until after 48 hours' incubation.

Anaerobic conditions may be produced conveniently by use of a modern cold-catalyst jar which is evacuated and filled with hydrogen —any remaining oxygen being eliminated by catalytic combination with hydrogen to form water. In using such jars to grow *Cl. tetani* it is useful to control the growth conditions as a matter of routine by ensuring that a stock culture of viable *Cl. tetani* does grow in the jar; in this way failure to achieve adequate anaerobiosis is clearly apparent.

Anaerobiosis suitable for growth of *Cl. tetani* may also be achieved in liquid media by means of reducing agents such as sodium thioglycollate, as in Brewer's medium, which also contains a little agar to impede gaseous diffusion. The addition of sterile iron strips to liquid media will also produce suitable reducing conditions. Liquid media should be heated for a few minutes in a boiling water bath before use in order to drive off dissolved oxygen; media should then be allowed to cool before inoculation. Probably the most convenient fluid medium for routine use is Robertson's cooked-meat broth. In using this medium it is necessary to ensure that it is provided in bottles giving a suitable depth of both the broth and the meat components; in McCartney bottles an adequate depth of medium is 6 cm, of which 3 cm is chopped meat.

On blood agar *Cl. tetani* does not usually form isolated colonies but appears as a fine, slightly granular film spreading over the whole plate—an appearance that is readily overlooked. If the swarm has not covered the whole plate its irregular rhizoid edge can be seen. Under the region of the initial inoculum the growth may be heaped up, and slight haemolysis is usually evident. This appears as a clearing of the blood, although some greenish discoloration may be evident in cultures examined after a short period of incubation. On agar plates that have been particularly well dried, defined, slightly haemolytic colonies may be formed which usually show one of three colonial appearances:

(i) a rhizoid colony, 2–4 mm in diameter;

(ii) a clear, lenticular colony about 1 or 2 mm in size with a spreading edge;

(iii) a cone-shaped colony, 1 mm in diameter.

By the incorporation of 3 to 4 per cent agar in the medium, isolated colonies can readily be obtained; they are more compact than those

seen on well-dried plates with a normal agar concentration.
Growth in liquid media occurs as a diffuse opacity, and in Brewer's thioglycollate medium the growth may have a fluffy appearance.

### *Biochemical activities*

*Cl. tetani* is inactive in the great majority of laboratory tests, having no action in peptone water-sugar media, apart from the occasional formation of a small bubble of gas which is attributed to breakdown of amino-acids in the peptone. Neither nitrates nor urea are attacked, although indole is produced from tryptophan and may be tested for in a peptone-water culture in the usual way with Ehrlich's reagent or by Kovacs' method. The species is not actively proteolytic so that cooked-meat broth cultures do not develop the mal-odour characteristic of the proteolytic clostridia such as *Cl. sporogenes* and many strains of *Cl. botulinum*. On the other hand the meat content of cooked-meat broth cultures is slowly affected and in old cultures the meat is reduced in volume and appears friable and darkened. Loeffler's serum slopes may show partial softening after *Cl. tetani* has been growing for 3 or 4 days. Gelatinase activity is present and is best tested for in gelatin medium incubated anaerobically at 37°C; liquefaction is detected by failure of the medium to solidify when removed from the incubator and allowed to cool—this may be hastened in the refrigerator or in running cold water. It is occasionally necessary to incubate the medium for as long as a week before gelatinase activity becomes evident.

The biochemical properties described above are those usually encountered in toxigenic *Cl. tetani*, but Nishida and his colleagues (see Nishida 1967) have recently described strains that attack glucose, others which form nitratase and, as might be expected, strains which do not attack tryptophan or gelatin.

### *Resistance*

The vegetative bacilli are no more resistant to adverse factors than other bacteria—they are readily killed by antiseptics and by heat. The spores, on the other hand, are highly resistant to antiseptics and fairly resistant to heat. Under suitable conditions—for example, in dried earth—the spores can survive for many years, although they are slowly killed in sunlight, provided air is present. One hour in water at 100°C usually suffices to kill spore preparations, but those of many strains are considerably less resistant, and heating in a boiling water bath for 5 minutes or even less will sterilize many spore suspensions. However, occasional strains are encountered with unusually resistant spores, and to ensure sterility 4 hours' boiling may be needed. In the autoclave at 121°C, tetanus spores are killed within ten minutes.

The spores are particularly resistant to antiseptics and can survive in 5 per cent lysol or 5 per cent phenol solution for as long as 2 weeks. The problem of chemical disinfection of tetanus spores was studied by Mackie (1928) in connection with the need to ensure the sterility of surgical catgut. He found the halogen antiseptics to be the most efficient; spores on the surface of catgut were killed by 1 per cent aqueous iodine within 3 hours. For sterilizing catgut, in which the spores may be protected, he recommended immersion in 1 per cent aqueous iodine solution for 7 days. Formaldehyde is not very active and spores can sometimes survive immersion in 2 per cent solution for up to 5 days. Recent evidence favours the use of 2 per cent glutaraldehyde at *p*H 7·5–8·5 (Rubbo & Gardner 1965) and our own experiments confirm the rapid killing effect of this preparation on *Cl. tetani* spores.

## *Toxins*

The two well-known toxins produced by *Cl. tetani* are tetanospasmin and tetanolysin.

*Tetanospasmin* is the highly potent neurotoxin that is the cause of the characteristic muscle spasm of tetanus. It is a typical bacterial exotoxin active in extremely small amounts—crystallized protein toxin can contain 50–75 million mouse lethal doses per milligramme (Pillemer *et al.* 1946). The fact that tetanus can be reproduced in experimental animals by injection of highly purified neurotoxin, and can be prevented by antitoxin specifically directed against that toxin, has led to the general acceptance that clinical tetanus is accounted for by the neurotoxin.

The amount of neurotoxin produced in culture varies appreciably with different strains of *Cl. tetani* and is also affected considerably by the nature of the growth conditions, and media have been devised that support a high toxin yield by suitable strains of bacilli (Mueller

& Miller 1954); such media are used in production of large quantities of toxin for conversion to toxoid vaccine. In the body tissue the amount of toxin which may be produced is not known with certainty. The amount must vary depending on the strain of tetanus bacilli and on the nature and extent of the anaerobic lesion, but it can be very large; thus, in guinea-pigs dying from infection with tetanus bacilli many thousands of mouse lethal doses of toxin can be found in the immediate vicinity of the infected lesion (Francis 1914).

*Tetanolysin* is the toxin responsible for the haemolysis seen on blood agar plates. It is active only in the reduced form, that is, under anaerobic conditions, and is therefore termed 'oxygen-labile'. Tetanolysin is closely similar in activity and in antigenic structure to the O-lysins produced by *Cl. welchii* ($\Theta$ toxin) and by streptococci of Lancefield groups A, C and G. It is doubtful whether tetanolysin has any important role in the pathogenic effect of *Cl. tetani*, but a toxic effect on leucocytes has been described.

An additional active fraction has recently been described in tetanus culture-filtrates by van Heyningen and his colleagues (Feigen *et al.* 1963). This factor has a peripheral action on the motor nerve endplate and may possibly be of some pathogenic importance, particularly in severely affected patients kept alive by curarization.

### *Antigenic structure*

Strains of tetanus bacilli have been divided into ten antigenic types by means of agglutination with antisera directed against the flagellar antigens, except in the case of Type VI, which is non-motile. A somatic 'O' antigen is common to all strains of *Cl. tetani*, but cross-reactions with an antigen present in *Cl. tetanomorphum* may be encountered. The spores have been described as possessing type-specific antigens different from those of the vegetative forms.

The neurotoxins (tetanospasmin) produced by each type of *Cl. tetani* are antigenically very similar, so that antitoxin prepared against toxin from one strain will neutralize toxin produced by any other strain.

The haemolysin (tetanolysin) is neutralized by specific antiserum and also by antisera to *Cl. welchii* $\Theta$ toxin and the O-lysin of *Strepto-*

*coccus pyogenes*. Antitoxin against tetanus neurotoxin usually contains some anti-tetanolysin activity.

## *Laboratory isolation of Cl. tetani*

(*a*) *Microscopy:* Examination of stained smears for the presence of typical drum-sticks of the sporing bacilli is most unreliable. Thus tetanus can very often be recovered by culture from material in which no typical organisms are to be seen and, moreover, typical drum-sticks are not necessarily toxigenic *Cl. tetani*.

(*b*) *Culture:* As with the isolation of any bacterium, the ease with which *Cl. tetani* can be grown from infected material depends on the number of bacilli present and on the number and nature of other bacteria which compete with it in culture. If tetanus bacilli are present in large numbers, direct plating of the source material on to blood agar will readily reveal the spreading colonies of *Cl. tetani* after 24 or 48 hours' anaerobic incubation. However, isolation is often more difficult and advantage must be taken both of spore formation and the tendency to swarm on agar surfaces. Culture of wound swabs is much less efficient than of pieces of tissue taken from the necrotic depths of the lesion, and it is, of course, essential that the correct material is examined—thus culture is more commonly successful when the material has been collected by an experienced surgeon. Pathological material should be cultured as soon as possible after collection, as vegetative *Cl. tetani* can die in air.

The material is distributed, depending on its quantity, into three bottles of cooked-meat broth medium and also plated on one half of a whole blood-agar plate in the hope that the swarming bacillus will spread to the opposite side of the plate after 1 or 2 days' incubation. In the case of soil or faeces, a convenient amount of material to be inoculated into the cooked-meat broth is about 1 g—which should be emulsified with sterile saline before addition to the culture medium. Isolation is facilitated from tissue if it is first cut into small pieces with sterile scissors or, better still, ground with sterile sand with a sterile pestle and mortar.

One of the cooked-meat broths should be heated to 80°C in a water bath for 15 minutes, one for 5 minutes, and the third left unheated. After heating, the broths should immediately be placed in a 37°C water bath in order to cool rapidly to the optimum growth temperature. The aim of the heating is to kill other bacteria whilst leaving tetanus spores undamaged. The different heating times are recommended because variation is encountered in the heat resistance of spores and also because the heat required to kill off the competing bacterial flora will vary according to its nature.

The cultures are then incubated at 37°C and subcultured on to one half of a whole blood agar plate daily for up to 4 days. These plates are incubated anaerobically and examined at 24 and 48 hours, particularly for the typical swarming edge of growth, but it should be remembered that non-motile strains do occur. The agar plates should not be exposed to the air for long and, with this in mind, some workers recommend that separate agar plates and anaerobic jars should be used for the 24- and 48-hour examinations. Recovery of the tetanus bacilli in pure culture is done by subculturing from the edge of the swarming growth. This may have to be repeated a number of times because the swarm can carry other bacteria with it.

If tetanus bacilli have not been isolated by the above procedure, success may occasionally be obtained by heating the incubated cooked-meat broths to 80°C and plating after 2, 5, 10, 20 and 30 minutes. This procedure may be essential if the culture contains *Proteus* species, the swarming of which can mask the swarming of *Cl. tetani*. It is also possible to use the cooked-meat broth cultures for further inoculation of fresh cultures both before and after heating, although this is not often successful when the previously-used procedures have failed.

Selective agar media have been devised for isolation of clostridia, including the tetanus bacillus, based usually on the presence of polymyxin B at a concentration of 2 mg per 100 ml, to which clostridia are resistant. Enrichment broths have also been used, e.g. sorbic acid—polymyxin B-thioglycollate broth (Wetzler *et al.* 1956).

It may be argued that for practical purposes the demonstration of *Cl. tetani* in a suspected source need not demand the isolation of a pure culture; all that is necessary is to show that the bacterial growth obtained from the material produces tetanus toxin (*vide infra*). Whilst this approach is not unreasonable, it must be pointed out that growth of *Cl. tetani*, or toxin production, may be inhibited by competing bacteria, and also that toxin may be destroyed by other bacteria. Consequently the absence of toxin in a mixed culture does not prove the absence of *Cl. tetani*. On the other hand, if toxin is demonstrated in a mixed culture the presence of *Cl. tetani* is implied.

Whilst, therefore, it is advisable to isolate *Cl. tetani* in pure culture whenever possible, it may often be worth while to test the primary cooked-meat broth cultures for the presence of toxin. The same argument applies to the attempted demonstration of toxin in pus or ground-up necrotic material taken directly from a wound; a positive result is acceptable, but a negative result does not mean that tetanus bacilli are not present, nor that the wound is not the origin of the tetanus.

### *Laboratory identification of Cl. tetani*

Identification of most bacteria depends on examination of the morphological, cultural, biochemical and, frequently, the antigenic properties of the strain. In the case of *Cl. tetani*, however, the test for tetanospasmin production is usually of overriding importance in clinical bacteriology. Nevertheless, it is good practice to test the principal properties of suspected strains. Thus, in addition to noting the morphological features, the absence of fermentative activity, the failure of strains to show much effect on cooked-meat broth, indole production and gelatinase activity should be confirmed. If it is desired to identify non-toxigenic strains of *Cl. tetani*, further tests, including agglutination reactions, may be necessary—for which the reader is referred to bacteriological text books.

The test for tetanospasmin must be done by demonstrating its specific biological effect in laboratory animals since no *in vitro* test for its presence has been established. The test is conveniently carried out by injecting 0·5 ml of a broth culture subcutaneously into the hind leg of a mouse. A cooked-meat broth culture that has been incubated for 48 hours usually contains sufficient toxin. An injection of culture is also given to a second mouse that has received an intraperitoneal injection of a large dose of antitoxin, e.g. 500–1000 units. (In tests of this sort, in which a whole culture is injected, a tetanus infection may be set up. The amount of horse antitoxin necessary to prevent tetanus in *infected* mice is large, and even 1500 units is occasionally insufficient.) If the broth contains tetanospasmin the unprotected mouse will develop ascending tetanus; stiffness is then first seen between 12 and 24 hours later in the leg in which the injection was made. At this stage the animal usually has some difficulty in turning over if it is placed on its back. The leg slowly becomes rigidly extended and the muscle spasm ascends to involve first the tail, which becomes erect and drawn to the injected side, then the opposite leg and, subsequently, the trunk, chest, front legs and neck. In the later stages, generalized reflex spasms are frequent and are induced by minor stimuli. The mouse usually dies within 48 hours, but the appearance of ascending tetanus is quite characteristic and as soon as the typical signs are recognized the mouse should be killed. The mouse protected with antitoxin almost invariably remains quite well, although when impure cultures are used the control animal may succumb to gas-gangrene caused by other clostridia in the inoculum.

An agar-plate identification procedure has been described by Lowbury and Lilly (1958) based on the neutralization of tetanolysin. This test employs horse blood agar plates prepared with 4 per cent agar to prevent swarming. Before use a few drops of ordinary commercial tetanus antitoxin (1500 units/ml) are spread over one half of the plate and allowed to dry. The suspected strain of *Cl. tetani* is stab-inoculated with a straight wire on each half of the plate which is then incubated anaerobically. Examination after 2 days shows, at each inoculation site, a compact granular colony with haemolysis apparent only around the colony on the half-plate not spread with antitoxin (ordinary antitoxin contains sufficient anti-tetanolysin to neutralize the haemolysin produced by the growing colonies.) Ten or twelve strains can conveniently be tested on one agar plate. There are, however, a number of possible objections to this technique. Thus, whilst the great majority of strains of *Cl. tetani* produce both toxins, the ability to produce tetanolysin is not always accompanied by tetanospasmin production. In addition, the O-lysins produced by streptococci and by *Cl. welchii* are antigenically very similar to tetanolysin and could possibly give rise to false-positive results, although none were found by Lowbury and Lilly. It is probably unwise to regard the procedure as a test of toxicity or virulence but rather as an additional laboratory test in the identification of *Cl. tetani*. It may be useful as an economical screening procedure for the recognition of suspected strains of tetanus bacilli isolated in survey work; the ability of strains identified in this way to produce neurotoxin should not be assumed but should be proved by an *in vivo* test.

The recognition of *Cl. tetani* in cultures, animal tissues, dressings, etc. can be done by means of fluorescent labelled antisera (Batty & Walker 1964). Whilst there is a possibility that false-positive results can occur owing to cross-reactions with common antigens shared with other bacteria, e.g. *Cl. tetanomorphum*, the available evidence suggests that this is not a practical problem and the method seems to be promising.

# 3

# THE DISEASE PROCESS

Tetanus, as its old German name 'Wundstarrkrampf' implies, in many cases follows wounding and can often be produced in experimental animals by the injection of earth. Since tetanus spores are widely distributed and can be found, for example, on clothing, all wounds are liable to be contaminated with *Cl. tetani.* Although it is probable that wounds frequently become contaminated with spores, tetanus rarely follows because the spores fail to germinate in the tissues; indeed the injection of washed tetanus spores into animals is usually followed by no ill-effects—the spores being phagocytosed and probably digested, although some can undoubtedly survive in the tissues for a number of weeks and perhaps occasionally for years (Bonney *et al.* 1938).

*Cl. tetani* is an anaerobe and in order to germinate and multiply, and produce neurotoxin, it requires a low oxygen tension. The healthy tissues are well oxygenated and have an oxidation-reduction potential (Eh) too high for germination to occur. Tetanus can follow contamination of a wound with spores only if an area with an Eh of less than +0·01 volts at *p*H 7·0 develops (Fildes 1929). Reducing conditions of this degree can arise in an area of necrosis such as may be produced by the presence of earth or calcium salts in the tissues; thus calcium chloride solution is commonly used for this purpose in the production of experimental tetanus in animals. Suitable conditions may also be produced by the growth of other bacteria infecting a wound, e.g. *Staphylococcus aureus.*

The growth of *Cl. tetani* is confined to the local anaerobic area, which may be extremely small, and yet this may lead to fatal tetanus on account of the extreme potency of the toxin. Tetanus bacilli can sometimes be cultured from parts of the body remote from the primarily infected site, but such organisms have probably escaped from the original focus of infection and are not multiplying. The growing bacilli produce neurotoxin (tetanospasmin) which is probably only released when autolysis occurs. The bacilli also release tetanolysin which may be responsible for the slightly haemorrhagic appearance that has been described around the local lesion.

In approximately 20 per cent of many series of cases of tetanus there is neither a history of injury nor a detectable wound (e.g. see Press 1948). In some areas a proportion of such idiopathic cases may be due to tetanus infection developing in a chronically infected middle-ear (otogenic tetanus), but the majority are probably accounted for by an injury which has gone unnoticed. Tetanus toxin is so highly potent that many lethal doses can readily be produced in a very small wound. Other idiopathic cases may possibly be accounted for by minor trauma at a site where tetanus spores have remained dormant after a previous wound. One of the commonest single causes of tetanus is infection occurring in the new-born infant when the raw umbilical stump becomes contaminated with spores. Other cases are attributable to infection of the genital tract post-partum and particularly after instrumental abortion. So-called 'endogenous tetanus' has also been described. It follows operation on the large intestine or gangrene of the bowel, the bacilli originating from the patient's own bowel. However, in whatever circumstances the disease develops the underlying pathological process is believed to be similar to that which occurs when the disease follows wounding.

The incubation period in human tetanus is variable—from 2 days to many weeks, although 6–12 days is the most commonly recorded period. Occasionally patients are seen with an incubation period of a number of months after an injury, but in such cases the possibility of a recent, unnoticed injury usually cannot be excluded. When the disease is produced in small laboratory animals by injecting spores suspended in calcium chloride, the incubation period is short—usually about 24 hours, and little variation is seen, even when the number of spores injected varies widely. In the experimental animal, therefore, spores germinate shortly after injection and it is possible that this is also true in man, in which case the long incubation seen in human tetanus must be attributed to the fact that, in man, toxin takes a long time to travel from the wound to the central nervous system. On the other hand it might be that anaerobic conditions develop slowly in the type of wound that gives rise to tetanus in man. Because, in man, the incubation period can sometimes be very short, and because it is so variable, the major factor affecting the incubation period is probably the nature of the wound itself. Thus, in some wounds anaerobic conditions develop rapidly and the spores germinate and multiply soon after injury so that the incubation period is short. In others, anaerobic conditions may not develop until some days or even weeks after injury, in which case the incubation period will be long.

The conditions at the site of infection must affect the severity of the disease as well as the incubation period. Thus the severity probably depends on the amount of toxin that reaches the central nervous system and on the rate with which it does so, and both factors must depend to a considerable extent on the amount and rate of toxin production in the wound. These factors in their turn presumably depend on the suitability of the conditions in the infected area for germination, growth and toxin production by the tetanus organisms, and also on the amount of toxin which the infecting strain can produce; different strains can have very different toxin-producing abilities. In view of these considerations, for which, it must be stated, there is little in the way of experimental evidence, it is not surprising that a valuable prognostic factor is the period of onset of the disease, i.e. the interval between the first symptom and the first reflex spasm—since this interval must be related to the amount and rate at which toxin is reaching the central nervous system.

### *Site of action and paths of spread of tetanus toxin*

It can now be taken as certain that the clinical picture of tetanus is virtually entirely due to the effects of toxin on the central nervous system and not on the peripheral nervous system or muscles, although toxin is not without some peripheral effect.

This conclusion has only been reached after prolonged dispute following experimental findings which were either susceptible of more than one explanation or could not be repeated by independent workers. Also, most of these studies employed the localized form of experimental tetanus, and Wright (1955) has pointed out that much disagreement has been the result of failure to appreciate that a muscle affected by experimental local tetanus passes through two stages (the stages are less clearly defined in generalized tetanus). The first, 'hypertonic contraction', lasting about 5 days, is characterized by profuse electrical activity which can be abolished by centrally and peripherally acting muscle relaxants, including general anaesthetics and curare, and by nerve section. In the second, or 'myostatic contracture' stage, the muscle remains contracted for weeks with diminished electrical activity and the contracture is unaffected by denervation or by muscle relaxants.

The myostatic contracture is unlikely to be due to a local action of the toxin. This is suggested by several facts: it follows the phase of hypertonic contraction, it can never be induced in denervated muscle and it occurs in muscles into which no toxin has been injected, but which are supplied by the same nerve roots. It may be that the intense continued contraction with shortening in the early stage causes changes in the muscle structure. Evidence on this is inconclusive, but it has been shown that contractures follow prolonged shortening of normal innervated muscle resulting from tendon section (Ranson & Dixon 1928), immobilization of approximated bony attachment points (Solandt *et al.* 1943) or continuous contraction due to motor activity induced by spinal cord anoxia (Gelfan & Tarlov 1959).

The evidence that the clinically important actions of toxin occur in the central nervous system and not on the peripheral nerve endings or muscles, and that toxin reaches the central nervous system by spread along peripheral nerves and by carriage in the blood, is now both voluminous and convincing.

Many of the experiments on these two topics throw light on both, so they will be treated together. The experimental evidence has been summarized by Laurence & Webster (1963) as well as by Wright (1955). Some of the most important items are given below.

1 Existing local tetanus is abolished by nerve section (Perdrup 1946). It could be argued that the toxin itself acts peripherally, modifying neuromuscular transmission, but depends on a functional innervation, and that experimental evidence only shows the need for this innervation. But there is evidence against this. Toxin has been found in the ventral, but not in the dorsal root (Kryzhanovsky 1966) and the following evidence also suggests a central action.

2 Denervation of a limb before or shortly after intramuscular injection of toxin stops the development of local tetanus (e.g. Hutter 1951). Section of the ventral motor root is effective whilst section of the posterior sensory root is not, indicating that toxin ordinarily travels into the anterior horn of the spinal cord where the motor cells lie.

Injection of toxin into the hind limb of one of a pair of parabiotic rats only induces local tetanus in the other if a crossed regenerated nerve is present (Schellenberg & Matzke 1958).

4 Injection of a very small dose of toxin into a nerve trunk is followed by spasm of all the muscles supplied by that nerve, however remote from the site of injection. Often the spasm spreads to the same segmental innervation on the opposite side of the body. Such experiments, first done in 1903 by Meyer and Ranson have since been repeated many times (Wright 1955) with extremely careful precautions to avoid leakage of toxin to the periphery.

A particularly elegant series of experiments is that of Wright *et al.* (1950) in which they showed that injection of toxin into the facial, vagus, or hypoglossal nerves is followed by strabismus, torticollis, salivation and bradycardia. With these experiments, leakage of the toxin to the periphery to affect all the organs involved might be thought impossible and, 'since the whole syndrome of bulbar tetanus is the same whether the toxin is injected into the facial, vagal or hypoglossal nerve, the simplest and most comprehensible explanation for these findings would seem to be that all these signs result from the central action of the toxin on these closely spaced brain stem nuclei whose neurones provide the final common pathway for the activation of these diverse effector organs' (Wright 1955).

5 Local tetanus in the hind limb of a rabbit is uninfluenced by occlusion of the arterial supply by an inflated cuff for one minute. However, a barbiturate given intravenously, so that it has access to the central nervous system but not to the leg, suppresses the electrical activity of the muscles within 15 seconds (Wright *et al.* 1952).

The above evidence is readily explicable by supposing that tetanus toxin acts centrally, and any hypothesis to explain it by a peripheral action puts an intolerable strain on credulity.

However, this does not mean that toxin is incapable of any peripheral effect, only that the central effects are responsible for most, if not all of the clinical picture. It has been shown that tetanus toxin injected into the anterior chamber of the rabbit eye will paralyse the cholinergic sphincter muscle of the iris (Ambache *et al.* 1948), and that on an isolated nerve-muscle preparation (mouse hemithorax), toxin 'raised the frequency of the random appearance of miniature end-plate potentials' (Feigen *et al.* 1963). The latter effect can be neutralized by antitoxin. Kryzhanovsky (1966) reports evidence of a decline in response of muscle to stimulation of the peripheral end of the cut motor nerve.

If tetanus toxin acts chiefly in the central nervous system, the question how it gets there from the site of infection deserves to be answered. This probably depends on where it is introduced into the body. The principal routes of transport are neural and vascular, the latter probably being the more important in generalized clinical tetanus.

Tetanus toxin in the gastrointestinal tract is absorbed in substantial amounts only if the lining mucosa is injured (Fedinec 1967).

*Nerve spread.* There is no doubt that toxin formed at or injected into the muscles or nerves can travel up the interstitial spaces of peripheral nerves at a rate of many millimetres an hour.

Intramuscular injection of a small dose of toxin into the hind limb of an animal causes a local tetanus confined to the segmental nerve supply at first on the same side, then on the opposite side and later spreading up the spinal cord to involve the whole body (ascending tetanus).

Important observations that demonstrate nerve transport of toxin, in addition to some of the experiments mentioned above, include the following:

1 If a zone of sclerosis is created by injection of an irritant chemical into the sciatic nerve of a rabbit then local tetanus does not follow the *distal* intramuscular injection of doses of toxin substantially greater than are needed to induce local tetanus in the absence of sclerosis; but typical local tetanus follows injection of the usual small amount of toxin into the nerve above (proximal) to the site of the sclerosis (Baylis *et al.* 1952).

2 Local tetanus following intraneural injection of toxin can be prevented by simultaneous injection of antitoxin into a proximal site on the ipsilateral nerve (Teale & Embleton 1920) and also if the antitoxin is injected into the contralateral nerve (Wright *et al.* 1951). This is achieved with doses of antitoxin which, given intravenously, will not prevent development of local tetanus (D'Antona 1951).

The notion that toxin passes up the motor axons themselves has had remarkably wide acceptance in the past, considering its intrinsic improbability and the total absence of any experimental support (Wright 1955). That the route by which the toxin travels centrally is the interstitial spaces of the nerves receives support from the nerve sclerosis experiments cited above as well as from the facts that other substances, such as dyes, India ink and radioactive isotopes, have been shown to pass up nerves, perhaps propelled by a current of tissue fluid resulting from the high pressures of muscular contraction (Wright 1953). Recent studies with tritium-labelled toxin confirm the route of spread described (Fedinec 1967). However, there is also evidence of flow of fluid in the opposite direction. Steer and Horney (1968) injected blue powder into the subarachnoid space of pigs and found it passed along peripheral nerves to the muscles. The exact anatomical path of toxin into the spinal cord needs further elucidation.

Spread of toxin up the spinal cord to the medulla has also been shown by experiments involving spinal section and antitoxin injections in the cord and by demonstration that radioactive isotopes pass rapidly upwards along the spinal cord in experimental animals (Wright 1955).

*Blood spread.* Toxin injected into animals intravenously causes tetanus that begins in the head, progressively and symmetrically involving the rest of the body from above (descending tetanus). When large doses of toxin are injected intramuscularly, not only does it pass up the motor nerves but some is also absorbed into the blood, providing a mixture of ascending (neural transport) and descending (blood transport) tetanus. Tetanus toxin injected subcutaneously enters the blood, probably not directly, but via the lymphatics, for toxin appears in the thoracic duct lymph before it does so in the blood, and immobilization of an injected limb by a plaster cast delays the onset of tetanus, although it does not delay the onset of the effects of strychnine which is absorbed directly into the blood. This difference can be explained by the fact that lymph flow is very largely dependent on muscular activity (it also increases with inflammation), whereas blood flow is much less so. It seems probable that the different routes of absorption of the toxin and strychnine are due to the differences in molecular weight, toxin being above 20,000 and strychnine below 400 (Barnes & Trueta 1941).

How toxin carried in the blood enters the central nervous system is not known. Wright (1955) suggests that, although in general the central nervous system capillaries are notably impermeable, there are areas, such as the *areae postremae* in the floor of the fourth ventricle, which 'permit the escape of substances from the blood with note-worthy ease'. He adds, 'it may be that this local capillary permeability in the floor of the fourth ventricle may, by permitting early intoxication of the nuclei of the lower cranial motor nerves, be responsible for the prompt involvement of the muscles of the jaw and neck in general tetanus'. However, studies with tritium-labelled toxin (Fedinec 1967) have not confirmed this.

There is also no explanation for the spread of toxin DOWN the cerebrospinal axis, it having been established that substances, including toxin, can pass UP this axis. Moreover, intravenous toxin can produce slight tetanus in the hind limbs of animals whose spinal cords have been cut (tetanus is always less after spinal section, supraspinal influences playing a part in maintaining cord activity). Although the possibility that toxin can pass out of all capillaries into the central nervous system in effective amounts has not been excluded it is necessary to consider an alternative possibility that at first meeting may seem bizarre.

Because the time between intravenous injection of toxin and death is inversely related to the size of experimental animal (Wright 1955), it has been suggested that toxin is transferred from the blood to the muscles and so to the central nervous system by transport up the peripheral nerves, as after intramuscular injection. If this were true it would also explain why the head is ordinarily affected before the limbs, for the march of events would depend on the length of the peripheral nerves.

Kryzhanovsky (1966) argues in favour of this explanation. There is, he contends, no true 'descending tetanus', i.e. toxin passing down the cerebrospinal axis; the appearance of the effects of tetanus toxin descending the spinal cord is simulated 'by the succession of toxin reaching the motor centers by neural pathways of different length—at first by the shortest (from muscles of the face and neck), then by longer ones (from muscles of the back) and so on'. The matter cannot be regarded as settled and further research must be awaited.

## *Mode of action of toxin*

The analogy between tetanus and strychnine poisoning has been drawn repeatedly since 1854. In 1909 Sherrington suggested that both substances abolished synaptic inhibition, and more recent work suggests that this occurs due to an action in the region of the anterior horn cells and related internuncial neurones (Brooks *et al.* 1957; Kryzhanovsky 1965). Initially polysynaptic reflexes are increased but monosynaptic are not, though they may be later on. Inhibitory influences on the spinal cord from centres in the brain and brain stem are reduced. Muscle rigidity and spasms occur throughout the body, agonists and antagonists contracting simultaneously because reciprocal inhibition is lost.

The clinical result of this abolition of inhibition is to induce a background of muscle rigidity, with spasmodic exacerbations elicited by a sudden stimulus entering the central nervous system. It may be supposed that the background rigidity, which does not occur with strychnine poisoning, is due to the exaggerated effects of the unavoidable minimum afferent input, including tonic proprioceptive impulses, acting on a spinal cord in which inhibitory influences are lacking. There is no evidence that the afferent input itself, e.g. from gamma neurones, is exaggerated in tetanus (Webster 1967).

If a rabbit with hind limb tetanus is placed in a sling and left quiet, the steady high level of electrical activity in the muscles declines slowly but increases immediately should the animal become restless or even a small afferent stimulus be applied, e.g. a tap on the frame supporting the sling. When developing assays of anticonvulsant drugs in tetanus, Laurence and Webster (1958) found that a stable background activity was best achieved by applying a small afferent stimulus once a minute.

Inevitably, the suggestion has been made that toxin prevents the release of an inhibitory neuro-transmitter in the spinal cord. Unfortunately the nature of any such transmitter is unknown, and the suggestion remains speculative. However, it has been shown that toxin is capable of preventing the release of a chemical transmitter, for, when injected into the anterior chamber of the eye, it prevents the release of acetycholine from the parasympathetic nerves to the iris (Ambache *et al.* 1948; Ambache & Mellanby 1965). Alternatively the toxin might block the effects of the inhibitory transmitter on the anterior horn cells by interfering with the receptor areas (Brooks *et al.* 1957). The prolonged duration of the effects of toxin (several weeks) implies that its action is to combine selectively with an important biochemical constituent. Van Heyningen and his colleagues (e.g. Mellanby & van Heyningen 1967) have studied the biochemical basis of tetanus toxin disposition in the central nervous system. They find that the toxin selectively combines with gangliosides (so does strychnine). As yet the significance of this in the development of the clinical state is uncertain and the practicability of interference with the toxin in the central nervous system as a therapeutic weapon is unexplored. The possibility that toxin exerts its effect by mediating production of a secondary substance is supported by some curious evidence that is otherwise hard to explain. Mice given 1 $LD_{50}$ of toxin 24 hours after receiving $\frac{1}{100}$ of this dose die sooner than others given the smaller dose only an hour previously (Janoff 1964; Mellanby & van Heyningen 1967).

There is also some evidence from the mode of death in cross circulation experiments and in parabiotic rats that supports this possibility (Schellenberg & Matzke 1958; Firor *et al.* 1940).

The fate of toxin bound in the central nervous system is unknown.

## *Physiological basis of the clinical picture of tetanus*

In man the classic, though not the invariable, presentation of tetanus is trismus, regardless of the site of the wound. This implies that toxin is carried by the blood and either enters the central nervous system in the region of the 5th nerve nucleus or, passing up all the motor nerves, affects the face first because these nerves are shortest (p. 24). Toxin travelling up the motor nerve supplying the area of toxin production will, if it is in an extremity, reach the central nervous system much later than if it is in the face, and any local intensification of tetanus at the site of wounding may be obscured by the concurrent appearance of generalized rigidity and spasms from blood spread. The disease is not always symmetrical, and during recovery it is not uncommon to detect differences which suggest that a wounded extremity has been the site of more intense muscle spasm than the others and has developed a noticeable myostatic contracture.

Whilst the tonic rigidity that is characteristic of clinical tetanus is probably maintained by the irreducible minimum of afferent stimuli entering the spinal cord and brain stem from the periphery, and spasms are superimposed when there are additional more vigorous stimuli, supraspinal influences such as emotion can also activate muscle spasm. In a case of tetanus selectively affecting both legs it was found that the knee-jerk could be elicited without precipitating spasm of the thigh muscles if the patient were calm, but the procedure was followed by vigorous spasm if the patient was agitated emotionally (Laurence 1957). This supports the acknowledged importance of careful nursing to reduce physical and emotional disturbance of the patient.

Local tetanus, usually in a limb or in the head and neck, though uncommon, is well recognized, and whilst it is probably more usual where passive immunization is practised, so that blood spread is prevented, it may occur in those who have no protection. Doubtless this is the result of the vicissitudes of toxin production in a wound whereby toxin passes up nerves from the site of injury with relatively little absorption into the lymphatics or blood. Sometimes local tetanus occurs initially and later becomes generalized whilst remaining more severe in the locally affected part. Local tetanus is easily produced in animals by intramuscular injection of a small dose of toxin. With larger doses generalized tetanus is produced because toxin also enters the blood. With these larger doses, however, generalized tetanus can be prevented by giving antitoxin intravenously in doses which do not prevent the development of local tetanus, for up to 80 times as much antitoxin is needed to neutralize toxin given intramuscularly (local nerve passage) than if that toxin is given intravenously (Friedmann *et al.* 1939).

In this connection it is of interest that what will probably remain the classic clinical account of local tetanus was written by Hurst (1944) from experience in the 1914–18 war. Here conditions resulted in a situation that crudely duplicated the animal experiments just mentioned. Large numbers of men were wounded under conditions where soil contamination was inevitable and copious, and immunoprophylaxis of tetanus consisted entirely of antitoxin given a variable time *after* wounding. In many cases enough time had elapsed to allow substantial toxin production. Blood-borne toxin was neutralized, but toxin nerve-borne from the site of injury was not (active immunization by toxoid was not introduced until 1927).

Whilst local tetanus may occur in the actively immunized, the presence of good immunity at the time of wounding may be supposed to render it less likely than when protection by antitoxin is only available later.

Rigidity is the predominant manifestation of local tetanus; reflex spasms occur but are generally not very prominent.

Early in local tetanus (hypertonic contraction), centrally or peripherally acting muscle relaxants or general anaesthesia will induce relaxation, but after a few days, when the myostatic contracture develops, they will not. Hurst (1944), discussing the differential diagnosis between tetanus and hysterical 'contracture', points out that an hysterical 'contracture' will always disappear under anaesthesia. Cases of the so-called 'stiff-man' syndrome have been diagnosed as local tetanus (*Brit. Med. J.* 1956) and the differentiation is most easily made from the prolonged history and the course of that disease.

### *Pharmacology of tetanus rigidity and spasms*

It has been pointed out (Laurence & Webster 1963) that if tetanus convulsions and spasticity result from exaggerated reflex response to afferent stimuli due to suppression of central inhibition, they may be controlled by drugs acting at different sites along the reflex pathway, as follows:

1 Hypnotics and sedatives, which reduce the effect of sensory input and the general state of excitability of the central nervous system. Barbiturates and paraldehyde are the classic examples.

2 General anaesthetics, which produce a widespread depression of the central nervous system.

3 Centrally-acting muscle relaxants which depress reflex activity and reduce motor output from the central nervous system. Mephenesin was the first of this group, which includes the phenothiazines (e.g. chlorpromazine) and the benzodiazepines (e.g. diazepam).

4 Peripherally-acting muscle relaxants, i.e. neuromuscular blocking agents, such as tubocurarine and gallamine.

The ideal of controlling rigidity and spasms without impairing respiration or voluntary movement is unattainable in severe cases with any drug or combination of drugs.

The less severe cases of tetanus can be treated with drugs from groups 1 to 3 above, but the most severe cases either cannot be controlled by them or can be controlled only with respiratory depression or loss of consciousness. Therefore in severe cases the most practicable course is, at present, to paralyse the patients completely with a neuromuscular blocking drug and to maintain pulmonary ventilation by mechanical means.

Attempts to use neuromuscular blocking agents in such a way

that they will reduce spasms whilst sparing respiration have had a little success, but the safety margin is small and respiratory failure is always imminent. Such use is not a practicable procedure even with gallamine which seems to have the greatest safety margin (Laurence & Webster 1963).

The site of action of an 'ideal' drug is likely to be central rather than peripheral, and the lack of an animal model on which tests could easily be made was a hindrance to any search. A technique of assessing antitetanus activity in the conscious animal was needed and was developed (Kelly & Laurence 1956) and refined (Laurence & Webster 1958*a*).

Local tetanus is induced in the hind limbs of rabbits by injecting toxin intramuscularly. It is then possible, using quantitative electromyography, to perform accurate comparative assays of drugs at the same time as observing their effects on respiration and consciousness. Antitetanus activity cannot be predicted by assaying activity against strychnine convulsions, for chlorpromazine is highly active against tetanus but not against strychnine convulsions. This fact throws doubt on the long-held belief that the effects on the central nervous system of strychnine and tetanus are identical. However, when strychnine is given in low doses that do not induce convulsions but merely exaggerate spinal reflexes, chlorpromazine may show some antistrychnine activity and this question therefore remains open (Laurence & Webster 1963). However, a stable state is more easily obtained with the toxin in addition to its advantage of being the actual disease-producing substance.

Using their technique, Laurence and Webster (1958*b*, 1961*a*) found that, apart from the suppressant activity of general anaesthetics and sedatives, phenothiazines were the most potent of a range of antitetanus agents that also spared respiration and consciousness. However, frequently repeated or single large doses had less or no effect and could even increase muscle activity (Laurence & Webster 1916). This apparent paradox probably results from the fact that the principal effect of chlorpromazine is in the brain-stem reticular formation which exerts both inhibitory and excitatory effects on the spinal cord; the phenothiazines interfere with the activity of both centres.

The mechanism of the antitetanus effect of phenothiazines is probably by reduction of both alpha and gamma motor nerve activity (Webster 1965). That there is also some effect directly on the spinal cord is shown by the fact that phenothiazines have a slight effect in tetanus in spinal animals (Webster 1962).

Despite the fact that large doses of phenothiazines can have the opposite effect to that which is desired, they are useful in clinical tetanus (see later) and are probably best used to a standard pre-determined dose schedule, for they cannot be 'titrated' against the muscle spasm as is the case with pure depressants such as barbiturates.

Mephenesin acts at both brain-stem and spinal levels, and is comparatively impotent. It reduces alpha motor neurone discharges only, in contrast to chlorpromazine which reduces both alpha and gamma neurone discharges. Since the clinical choice of drugs for conservative treatment of tetanus is not critical, it would not be useful to go into the minutiae of drug differences and modes of action found in the laboratory; in any case the latter are largely speculative. For more detailed discussion see Laurence and Webster (1963) and Webster (1965).

The most effective drugs that do not induce unconsciousness are the phenothiazines, diazepam and mephenesin.

The action of mephenesin is so brief and the effective dose is so large as to render its routine use almost impracticable. Diazepam is both more potent and several times longer-acting than mephenesin. The phenothiazines are highly potent and long-acting (see also p. 116).

Of those drugs that induce unconsciousness, the barbiturates are the most important.

# 4
# EPIDEMIOLOGY

Tetanus kills a great many people and is a major public health problem in most developing countries (Veronesi 1967). Accurate figures for morbidity and mortality are not available because it is not a notifiable disease in about half the countries in the world and because it is commonest where arrangements for collecting health data are least developed. However, it is likely that total world deaths exceed 160,000 per annum and, if the crude case fatality is taken as about 45 per cent, there must be about 355,000 cases. The crude case fatality rate (all ages) in different areas is very variable, from 40 to 70 per cent (Bytchenko 1967); it probably depends on numerous factors such as the soil, type of wound and availability of medical care, as well as the attitudes of the local population to injury and to illness.

Tetanus is more common where the climate is warm, and in rural areas where the soil is fertile and highly cultivated, the population of man and animals is substantial and there is a low material standard of living. The crucial factors seem to be: a liability to physical injury (as in agricultural labourers who work barefoot on soils where the clostridia are plentiful); lack of material facilities and education to prevent and treat sepsis; lack of effective programmes of active immunization. Seasonal variations occur, generally in the direction of more tetanus in hot weather, but they are not very great.

Striking differences in incidence occur in neighbouring areas. For example, amongst the African population of Lesotho, where the climate is dry, tetanus is virtually unknown, whereas in that of neighbouring Natal, lower lying and humid, it is common. Another possible explanation may be that there are important differences in soil cultivation.

The relationship between the distribution of *Clostridium tetani* in the soil with tetanus morbidity and climate has been studied by Sergeeva and Matveer (1967) who examined 5338 soil samples in the U.S.S.R. They found the soils with highest contamination were those in the fertile, warm regions, particularly where the human and animal populations were also high. Tetanus morbidity was also maximal in these areas and has been reduced 4 to 6 times by programmes of active immunization. In Moscow 3 per cent of soil samples contained *Cl. tetani* but in rural areas contamination was as high as 33 per cent. Other studies give figures for contamination of soil or dust in temperate cities from 12 to 55 per cent. Clearly, whilst wounds acquired in rural areas may be particularly heavily contaminated, there is also definite risk in modern cities. Tetanus following trivial wounds in these cities is well recognized though not as common as in rural areas.

The fact that the incidence of the disease was declining in Europe, U.S.A., Japan and Australia before the introduction of tetanus toxoid suggests that the standard of living and urbanization are important.

The reported increase in tetanus in some developing tropical countries is probably chiefly due to improving registration practices, to the spread of effective health services and to the growth of confidence in them by the population (Bytchenko 1967) and so is apparent rather than real. It points to the futility of erecting complicated structures of interpretation on the available figures. That these can be extremely inaccurate is shown by the fact that from some Central and South American countries the number of deaths reported is about twice the number of registered cases (Bytchenko 1967); registration of death is more likely to be reliable than registration of sickness.

The range in mortality is enormous. In African countries it varies between 0·1 and 135·0 per 100,000 inhabitants per annum. In North America the range is 0·06 to 0·18 and in Central and South America it is 0·7 to 63·3.

Despite the inadequacy of epidemiological statistics it is likely that mortality from tetanus is generally declining throughout the world as the following examples (Table 4.1) of decennial mortality rates per 100,000 inhabitants suggest (Bytchenko, 1967).

Crude case fatality rates do not give an accurate overall picture, for tetanus neonatorum carries a particularly high rate, almost always above 80 per cent in the absence of the most modern facilities for treatment. Adult fatality rates are more often 20 to 50 per cent. Tetanus neonatorum can also be an extremely important cause of neonatal death, accounting for up to 70 per cent of such deaths in

TABLE 4.1

| Country | Years 1921–30 | Years 1951–60 |
|---|---|---|
| New Zealand | 0·87 | 0·45 |
| Mauritius | 10·48 | 9·56 |
| Denmark | 2·49 | 0·34 |
| Canada | 0·49 | 0·06 |
| Ceylon | 5·48 | 3·51 |
| Japan | 4·77 | 1·05 |
| U.S.A. | 1·20 | 0·18 |
| England and Wales | 0·38 | 0·09 |

less developed countries. It is extremely rare where a high standard of obstetric hygiene is established routine. That climate is relatively unimportant, compared with hygiene, is suggested by the fact that in the late 18th century tetanus was responsible for the death of 30 per cent of new-born infants in parts of temperate Scotland. Fifty years later the disease had disappeared and the disappearance was attributed, doubtless correctly, to elimination of 'unskilful treatment on the part of self-taught midwives' (see also p. 37). Recent figures from Japan confirm this: improving obstetrical facilities were accompanied by a drop in neonatal tetanus deaths from 36 to 7 per cent (Ebisawa 1967).

Tetanus affects males more often than females, generally in a ratio of 2 or 3 to 1, but sometimes more, perhaps because male activities result in more injuries. However, there is a preponderance of males with tetanus neonatorum in some areas, and this plainly cannot be explained on that basis; Martin-Brouyer (1967) and Suri (1967) make the disheartening suggestion that the reason is that female infants are so little regarded in some of the less developed communities that parents do not trouble to obtain medical attention and they die unrecorded.

Unfortunately, substantial numbers of cases of tetanus have occurred as a result of medical and surgical interventions. Often these follow frankly dirty procedures by non-professionals, e.g. circumcisions, ear-piercing*, abortions, ritual incisions, etc., or the application of soil, ashes, dung to wounds and the umbilicus.

* In Dakar (Senegal) ear-piercing is responsible for 34 per cent of cases of tetanus in girls (Rey *et al.* 1967).

However, cases also occur following professional treatments, such as injections (particularly intramuscular quinine which causes muscle necrosis), vaccination for smallpox and tuberculosis and any surgical operation.

These must be attributed to failures of technique at the time of the intervention or in its aftercare. Heredia (1965) reports an average of 5 post-operative cases of tetanus per annum from 1954 to 1962 in a large Bombay hospital group doing more than 20,000 operations of all kinds per annum. He remarks that it is usual to fail to find the source of infection in cases of surgical tetanus, but attributes them to the ubiquity of *Cl. tetani* as a result of the substantial population of cattle and horses, even in the centre of the city, and to failures of sterilization of instruments, dressings or sutures, or to their contamination in bad storage conditions after sterilization. These failures are ordinarily due to economic difficulties. Heredia advocates active immunization of patients awaiting major 'cold' surgery by 3 toxoid injections in one month wherever post-operative tetanus is endemic.

Where post-surgical tetanus is not a continuing hazard there may yet be sporadic outbreaks. In one such outbreak (Mackay-Scollay 1959) 5 cases occurred in patients operated on in three theatres during 5 days. The theatres were closed at once, intensively cleaned, and all patients who had been operated on during that and the previous week were given 50,000 I.U. of antitoxin.

An intensive investigation included examination of dust and debris from furniture, walls (surface and from drillings), floors and the ventilating system. 'Tetanus spores were found widely distributed throughout the theatre block: from all floors of the theatres, the anaesthetic room, the main corridor, sluice and surgeons' changing room. *Cl. tetani* was also isolated from the broken plaster in the wall of the annexe corridor, the wall of the anaesthetic room, the light over Theatre I operating table and the light bulb in the packing room,' as well as from the ventilating system and the outside roof near to the ventilation exhaust. 'Undoubtedly the vigorous cleaning efforts, which had been put in hand when the theatres were closed, had contributed to the wide dissemination; but it is worth noting that spores were found readily despite these decontamination processes.'

Sutures, dusting and therapeutic powders, instruments and gloves were all examined. Some gloves were found to be contaminated. Since there had been no change in packing or sterilizing technique it was necessary to consider why this particular contamination should have occurred. It was eventually concluded that the gloves had probably been infected from a particularly septic amputation that had taken place in one theatre about 2 weeks before the first case of tetanus. Proof of the source of post-operative tetanus is particularly difficult because the investigation cannot begin until the disease has declared itself. In these cases the average incubation period was 6 days.

Lowbury and Lilly (1958) found tetanus spores in 89 per cent of samples of air outside a hospital in a large city (Birmingham, England), in 65 per cent of samples in an exhaust ventilated operating theatre, but none in the air of a dressing station ventilated with filtered air. They comment that post-operative tetanus had not occurred for 9 years in that hospital and conclude that an unusual increase in amount of spores is probably needed to induce infection.

Post-operative tetanus is rare after rectal operations, despite the relative frequency of *Cl. tetani* in human faeces. The fact that post-operative tetanus usually occurs in small outbreaks rather than in single cases indicates that self-infection is less important than environmental infection.

It has long been believed that infection at certain sites, such as the face and head, causes a particularly high mortality. This is probably untrue, except perhaps in the case of tetanus arising in the genital tract (see p. 95). Puerperal tetanus is commoner after instrumental abortion than after labour at full term. The reported fatality rate is high, from 50–90 per cent, but it is not certain to what extent this is influenced by the social circumstances surrounding abortion rather than by the characteristics of the site of infection. Substantial series of cases are now no longer reported.

Tetanus from ear-piercing (Rey *et al.* 1967) and from otitis media (Vakil *et al.* 1965; Patel *et al.* 1965; Suri 1967) is said to carry a particularly low mortality.

# 5

# PREVENTION OF TETANUS I

The pathological process in tetanus offers a number of points at which intervention might be successful in preventing the disease. Thus the introduction of spores into the tissues can to some extent be prevented by measures that reduce the frequency of injuries, for example, the wearing of shoes. When wounding does occur, dirt, foreign matter and dead tissue can be removed by surgery, which cannot only remove spores but, by promoting healthy healing, may also prevent the development of conditions suitable for spore germination. If these measures are judged to be insufficient, chemoprophylaxis can be employed to render harmless any spores which may remain in the tissues. Alternatively, the patient can be provided with the means of neutralizing any toxin that might be formed in a wound by giving him an injection of antitoxin-rich serum, obtained either from immune animals or from other persons who have been immunized. It is also possible to provide long term and very effective resistance to tetanus by means of active immunization with tetanus toxoid.

All these methods of prophylaxis are in use and they are discussed according to the stage in the pathological process with which they interfere. It should be pointed out, however, that there is great difficulty in assessing the value of many of the prophylactic procedures because tetanus follows injuries so rarely. In Ibadan (Nigeria) the incidence of tetanus among patients treated for injury in the casualty department of University College Hospital was 4·34 per 10,000 (Lucas & Willis 1965), and in India, where tetanus is common, less than 1 in 7000 of wounded patients seen in casualty departments develop the disease. No properly controlled field study to assess the value of any of the prophylactic methods has been carried out in man, and such studies would need to be done on a very large scale in order to provide valid results. It must be appreciated, therefore, that many of the statements made about the various preventive measures are based on clinical impressions and on animal experiments, neither of which are substitutes for properly controlled clinical trials.

### *Prevention of wound contamination*

Measures that prevent injuries and which decrease contamination of wounds are of major importance in preventing tetanus and there are a number of examples which may be used to illustrate the importance of this approach. These include the decline in the incidence of tetanus which followed the discouragement of the use of blank cartridges in the 4th of July celebrations in the U.S.A. in the early years of this century, and, also, the importance of careful sterilization of surgical catgut in prevention of post-operative tetanus (Mackie 1928). A particularly good example of the importance of general hygienic measures concerns *tetanus neonatorum* on the island of St. Kilda, Scotland. In the 19th century this disease caused the death of about half of the babies born on the island; the introduction of hygienic precautions in the care of the umbilical stump, together with the use of antiseptics, eliminated the disease (Turner 1895).

Hygienic precautions are particularly relevant to the prevention of tetanus today. A great part of human tetanus occurs among new-born infants in developing countries owing to the poor hygiene practised by untrained midwives—indeed, in many parts of the world material such as cow dung is deliberately applied to the umbilical stump, sometimes for ritual purposes. There is no doubt that elimination of such practices, together with the adoption of proper hygienic midwifery, can have a marked influence on the incidence of tetanus.

### *Surgical prophylaxis*

Clearly many wounds will occur and become contaminated, despite hygienic precautions, and prophylaxis may then be attempted by surgical means. The aim of surgery is the removal of all dirt and foreign matter, the excision of dead and dying tissue, and the promotion of healing with healthy, well-oxygenated tissues in which no dead spaces occur. These measures remove spore-carrying material from the wound and prevent the formation of anaerobic foci in and around foreign bodies, dead tissue and infected pockets. It must be emphasized, however, that all wounds are liable to be contaminated with tetanus spores even if there is apparently no dirt or soil in the wound because of the wide distribution of the spores in the environment.

The importance of surgical débridement and cleaning in preventing tetanus is often emphasized (e.g. see Edsall 1959), but it is interesting to note that very little evidence of its value exists. Wide surgical excision of wounds was introduced into the treatment procedures for British soldiers during World War I. When this was done the incidence of tetanus among soldiers returned to Britain after being wounded in France fell from 103 to 24 per 100,000 (Bruce 1920). This fall has been attributed to the surgical measures, but it could be argued that some other, unrecognized change in the circumstances of wounding was responsible, for appreciable fluctuations in the incidence of tetanus in wounded soldiers occurred throughout the war. McDonald *et al.* (1960) attempted to prevent the development of tetanus in experimentally infected guinea-pigs by surgical excision of the entire muscle mass into which spores in calcium chloride had been injected; they failed. In these experiments, however, 8 hours were allowed to elapse between injection of the spores and the surgical excision, and it is possible that a lethal dose of toxin had already been produced by this time.

Despite the absence of sound field or laboratory evidence of the value of surgical measures, a knowledge of the pathological process indicates that surgical cleaning of the wound is likely to be an important factor in preventing tetanus and its effectiveness cannot seriously be doubted. Surgery must therefore form an important part of any prophylactic scheme for tetanus prevention in wounded patients; indeed, débridement forms part of the normal wound care procedure and is practised irrespective of measures which aim specifically at preventing tetanus.

In the majority of the prophylactic schemes that have been published, it is suggested that surgical measures suffice for prophylaxis in superficial wounds which can be completely cleaned, provided the patient is seen within a few hours of injury. A time limit is set because a lethal dose of toxin may already have been formed in a wound which is treated late, in which case surgery could not prevent the disease. This is undoubtedly a reasonable view to take and is justified by experience, but the time period after wounding for which surgical cleaning can be considered sufficient must be decided arbitrarily. Six hours is suggested as reasonable, since there is some evidence that a lethal dose of toxin can be formed after this time in experimentally-infected animals (Smith 1964).

In many discussions on tetanus prophylaxis, special consideration is given to the 'tetanus-prone' wound, by which is meant a wound particularly likely to have been contaminated by tetanus spores under conditions in which they could germinate. Such wounds are those contaminated with soil and manure; wounds in which foreign bodies or dead muscle may be retained; deep puncture wounds in which surgical cleaning is difficult or impossible; and wounds seen late after injury (e.g. more than 6 hours), when tetanus toxin may already have been produced or pyogenic infection already be established. It seems very likely that such wounds are particularly liable to give rise to tetanus, although we know of no controlled field evidence clearly substantiating this view. On the other hand, it has been argued that all wounds should be regarded as 'tetanus-prone' on the grounds that in many series of cases tetanus often follows unnoticed or very minor injuries. Since in the areas from which such series are reported the majority of severe injuries receive some form of tetanus prophylaxis, it is to be expected, if the prophylaxis is effective, that severe wounds should contribute to only a small proportion of the clinical tetanus seen. From a knowledge of the pathological process it is clearly realistic to regard wounds such as those described above as 'tetanus-prone': the patient severely injured by a tractor in a farm-yard requires a more extensive prophylactic regimen than the patient who cuts his finger whilst opening a clean tin in a clean kitchen.

## *Chemoprophylaxis*

Bacteria and dead tissue may remain in a wound despite surgical measures, and there is no doubt that germination of tetanus spores may occur and lead to fatal tetanus in patients whose wounds have been apparently thoroughly cleaned. Chemoprophylaxis aims at inhibiting multiplication of such organisms, and if possible killing them, so that the production of toxin is prevented.

In experimentally infected animals, tetanus can be prevented by chemoprophylaxis under limited conditions. As in the case of surgical measures, antibiotics fail to prevent tetanus once a lethal dose of toxin has been produced (tetanospasmin is unaffected by antibiotics). Thus chemoprophylaxis was found to be effective in mice at 4 hours after infection, but not at 8 hours; presumably toxin had already formed by this time (Smith 1964). It is difficult to decide how such experimental findings should be related to prophylaxis of human tetanus because the incubation period in man is often about 10 days, whereas in experimental animals it is usually about 24 hours. As discussed earlier (p. 18), the long incubation period in man may well reflect that conditions suitable for the germination of spores often do not develop until late after injury, in which case chemoprophylaxis, and also surgical measures, should be effective even if delayed until several days after an injury. However, since the incubation period in man is sometimes very short, and because a number of failures of antibiotic prophylaxis have been reported in which treatment was not started until late after injury, it is probably wisest not to rely on chemoprophylaxis in patients seen later than about 6 hours after wounding.

The experimental work also shows that tetanus organisms can survive in the tissues despite a prolonged course of an antibiotic to which they are sensitive. The effectiveness of antibiotics can probably be partly explained by their ability to prevent multiplication of the bacilli until such time as the lesion is no longer anaerobic. Consequently, in providing an antibiotic for tetanus prophylaxis it should be given until the lesion has ceased to be anaerobic. Unfortunately, it is not known for how long anaerobic conditions may last in the various types of lesion in man in which tetanus bacilli grow—the only guide is from animal experiments. In guinea-pigs injected with non-toxigenic spores in calcium chloride, Russell (1927) showed that the organisms germinated, multiplied and resporulated within 5 days. It has also been shown in mice injected with toxigenic spores in calcium chloride, that a 4-day course of penicillin suffices to prevent tetanus, even though *Cl. tetani* can be recovered from the injection site subsequently (Smith 1964). These observations suggest that the experimental calcium chloride lesion remains anaerobic for about 4 days, but unfortunately it cannot be claimed that anaerobic lesions in man also last for only 4 days. Since the animal work is the only evidence available, it is probably wise in using antibiotic prophylaxis in man to provide at least a 4-day course—shorter periods are insufficient in mice and may be insufficient in man. Because tetanus organisms can survive in the tissues despite a course of penicillin, it is necessary to continue antibiotics for longer periods if wound healing is delayed and there is a possibility that anaerobic areas might persist or redevelop. Tetanus could presumably develop late after injury in patients given chemoprophylaxis, just as it did in soldiers given horse antitoxin in World War I (Bruce 1920).

The concentration of antibiotic that must be maintained in the serum in order to protect cannot be determined with certainty. It has been found that 0·1 unit of free penicillin per ml is adequate to prevent tetanus in mice injected with penicillin-sensitive *Cl. tetani* suspended in calcium chloride and, in the absence of further information, this level should probably be regarded as the minimum for protection. It is possible, however, that antibiotic may penetrate less freely into the sort of area in which *Cl. tetani* might grow in naturally-occurring wounds, e.g. a piece of dead, soiled tissue, and because of this doubt chemoprophylaxis should not be relied upon in wounds from which dead tissue and foreign material cannot be removed. There is evidence that the injection of antibiotic into or near the site of infection can be more effective than when it is injected elsewhere (Novak *et al.* 1949; McDonald *et al.* 1960), presumably owing to the higher concentration achieved in the vicinity of the bacilli. The local application of antibiotic powder to the wound when the surgical débridement is done should therefore be considered as a useful prophylactic measure.

An additional point of importance is the question of chemoprophylaxis in contaminated wounds. Thus penicillin reaching a wound may be inactivated by penicillinase produced by staphylococci and other bacteria growing in the wound, so that tetanus bacilli, which do not produce penicillinase, can be protected from the antibiotic. In obviously contaminated wounds it is wisest to use antibiotics other than benzyl penicillin, e.g. cloxacillin, erythromycin or tetracycline.

In addition to the laboratory experiments there is also a limited amount of field evidence which suggests that chemoprophylaxis can be effective in non-immune wounded patients who are thought to require a prophylactic measure in addition to careful surgical cleaning. Thus some centres have abandoned the use of horse serum antitoxin in favour of antibiotics, and no increase in the incidence of tetanus among the treated patients has been reported from two of these centres (Filler & Ellerbeck 1960; Cox *et al.* 1963). On the other hand there are a number of published examples of patients who developed tetanus despite chemoprophylaxis, e.g. the report of Lucas and Willis (1965) from Ibadan, Nigeria. However, in a number of these patients chemoprophylaxis should not have been relied upon, for example, when the patients were seen later than 6 hours after injury, and in others the antibiotic may have been given for too short a time.

Although chemoprophylaxis can probably be a reliable and effective procedure if properly used, a point of considerable importance is the antibiotic sensitivity of *Cl. tetani*; clearly if drug resistance is common, antibiotics cannot be used for preventing tetanus. Very little information exists on this point. As might be expected, dormant spores are resistant except possibly to very high concentrations of penicillin (Scheibel & Lennert-Petersen 1958; Anwar & Turner 1956), but it seems probable that tetanus bacilli are usually sensitive to many antibiotics. Results of the few small surveys that have been made (Scheibel & Assandri 1961; Lindberg & Newton 1954; Garrod 1958; Smith 1964; Lowbury 1967) suggest that *Cl. tetani* is usually sensitive to the penicillins, erythromycin and tetracycline, although strains resistant to penicillin and to chloramphenicol have been described. Resistance to streptomycin is common and all strains are resistant to polymyxin B—advantage of this is taken in the preparation of selective media. If antibiotic prophylaxis is to be used in a particular region it may be advisable to conduct a local survey to ensure that strains of *Cl. tetani* present in the soil of the locality are sensitive to the antibiotics it is proposed to employ.

When an antibiotic is to be given for prophylaxis it is necessary to decide not only which antibiotic to give, but also how it should be given. Penicillin, cloxacillin, erythromycin and tetracycline can all be given orally, but patients with minor injuries may not continue to take their prescribed tablets for more than a day or two and for this reason many surgeons feel that the antibiotic should be given by injection. Procaine penicillin G can be injected intramuscularly twice daily to provide adequate blood levels, but this is unlikely to be acceptable unless the patient is in hospital, and a single injection of a large dose of benzathine penicillin may be preferred. When benzathine penicillin is given it is probably advisable to use a preparation which also contains benzyl and procaine penicillin to ensure that an adequate blood concentration of antibiotic is present in the hours immediately following the injection, e.g. a mixture of benzathine penicillin, 1 g, procaine penicillin, 600 mg, and benzyl penicillin, 380 mg. The 1 g-dose of benzathine penicillin should provide an adequate blood penicillin concentration for 4 days (Tinkler & Shannon 1966).

The place of antibiotics in prophylactic schemes cannot, at the present time, be finally decided. In developed countries, where medical care is of a high standard and the majority of patients are seen shortly after wounding, chemoprophylaxis is probably an acceptable alternative to antitoxin prophylaxis for most patients. A major factor in deciding which procedure to employ must be an assessment of the relative incidence of hypersensitivity reactions to antibiotics and to horse serum antitoxin in the area concerned. Thus in Britain and the U.S.A. the incidence of hypersensitivity reactions to horse serum, in patients giving no general reaction to a trial dose, has been estimated to be from 5 to as much as 50 per cent by different workers. In India, on the other hand, the incidence appears to be low—of the order of 2·5 per cent in patients giving no general or local reaction to a trial dose (Patel *et al.* 1965). The incidence of hypersensitivity reactions to antibiotics is not known with certainty, but in the case of penicillin it has been estimated to be between 0·7 and 10 per cent in the general population (Idsøe *et al.* 1968), that is, appreciably lower than the incidence of horse-serum hypersensitivity in Britain.

# 6

# PREVENTION OF TETANUS 2

## *Prophylaxis by immunization*

Tetanus can be prevented by neutralizing the toxin released from an infected site before it can reach the central nervous system. This may be achieved either by active immunization, which stimulates the patient to form his own circulating antitoxin, or passive immunization, in which antitoxin is provided for the patient in the form of purified immune serum obtained from an animal or from other immunized men.

*The potency of antitoxic serum* is assessed in international units by comparing its toxin-neutralizing activity with that of the International Standard Tetanus Antitoxin which is held for the World Health Organization at the International Laboratory for Biological Standards, Statens Seruminstitut, Copenhagen. Suitable antitoxins that have been titrated against the International Standard are issued by national laboratories so that workers all over the world are able to assess the potency of antisera in terms of international units.

The titration procedure consists of determining the amount of antiserum that has the same neutralizing power as a known amount of standard antitoxin. A series of mixtures is prepared, each containing the same amount of standard tetanus antitoxin, e.g. 1/100th unit, together with different amounts of a test preparation of tetanus toxin. Each of the mixtures is injected into groups of mice, and the animals are carefully observed in order to determine the amount of toxin which, when mixed with the known amount of antitoxin, causes the mice, on average, to die of tetanus on the fourth day. This amount of toxin is called the test dose. If the known amount of standard antitoxin used is 1/100th unit, then the test dose is called the L+/100 dose. Dilutions of the unknown serum are then mixed with the test dose of toxin and injected into groups of mice. The mixture that allows the mice to die, on average, on the fourth day, contains the same amount of antitoxin (e.g. 1/100th unit) as was used in the preliminary titration with standard antitoxin.

Antitoxin may also be tritrated by haemagglutination of red cells that have been sensitized with tetanus toxoid. When the unitage is determined in this way the result is not necessarily the same as that obtained from measurements in animals, probably because some of the antibodies reacting in haemagglutination are against impurities in the toxoid, whilst others are antibodies capable of combining with the toxin molecule without neutralizing its toxic activity. Somewhat better correlation may be obtained by means of haemagglutination-inhibition tests (Fulthorpe 1957).

The amount of tetanus antitoxin needed in the circulation in man in order to prevent tetanus cannot be measured directly, and even in animal experiments its assessment presents problems. Thus the protective effect of a given serum antitoxin concentration must depend on such variable factors as the amount of toxin formed in an infected wound and the rate at which it is released. Nevertheless, mainly on the basis of animal experiments, the 'protective' concentration has been variously estimated at from 0·001 to 0·2 units per ml, and in recent years there has been a tendency to accept 0·01 units per ml as adequate (Tasman & Huygen 1960; Edsall 1959; McComb & Dwyer 1963). This view is supported by the work of MacLennan and his colleagues (MacLennan *et al.* 1965), who found that when pregnant women were actively immunized to provide a mean serum antitoxin concentration in the last trimester of 0·01 unit per ml, tetanus was prevented in their newborn infants by the resulting passive immunity.

## *Passive immunization*

Passive immunization aims at providing a protective amount of antitoxin in the serum of the injured patient over the period of time for which toxin formation might occur in a wound. Prophylaxis by the injection of tetanus antitoxin prepared in another animal was first used in the field as early as 1897, when Nocard showed that injections of antitoxic horse serum prevented tetanus in horses subjected to surgery (Nocard 1897). In man, passive immunization has been practised on a world-wide scale since World War I, using horses, almost entirely, to provide the large quantities of antitoxin required. The animals are carefully immunized first with toxoid and later with increasing doses of toxin, until their blood is extremely rich in antitoxin—it is not uncommon for donor horses to yield serum containing 1000 units of antitoxin per ml.

In most countries crude horse serum has been replaced by 'refined' antitoxin in which the antitoxic globulin of the whole serum has been purified and concentrated by digestion with pepsin and by salt and heat precipitation. Digestion probably acts by splitting off that part of the globulin antibody molecule which carries most of the species-specific antigenicity, and this fraction can then be removed by heat precipitation (Pope 1963; Porter 1963). The process of refining yields a relatively concentrated product of considerably diminished antigenicity for man; in consequence, this provokes hypersensitivity reactions less frequently than crude horse serum and is less liable to immune elimination (*vide infra*).

When antitoxin is injected into the animal body it is, like other proteins, first distributed through the blood and tissues. This process may be slow if the protein is injected intramuscularly or subcutaneously. The serum concentration then falls steadily as the protein disappears from the blood and is broken down. The half-life of protein in the blood during this catabolic phase of elimination varies from about 1 to 12 days according to the nature of the protein and the species of animal; in the case of homologous proteins the half-life is usually longer (Weigle 1957). Following the catabolic phase of elimination a phase of rapid, immune elimination usually supervenes in the case of foreign proteins (Glenny & Hopkins 1922). This phase is a result of the development of antibodies that combine with the foreign antigen and cause its rapid removal from the circulation and breakdown in the tissues, a process which may be accompanied by a hypersensitivity reaction, serum sickness.

If the injected animal has had previous experience of the foreign protein, antibodies may develop very quickly (a secondary antibody response), with the result that the immune phase of elimination starts much sooner than in the normal animal, and may be accompanied by accelerated serum sickness (Dixon *et al.* 1951). If circulating antibodies against the foreign protein are already present at the time of injection, the immune phase of elimination will start immediately and may be accompanied by anaphylaxis (Francis *et al.* 1957). In these circumstances the protection provided by injected antitoxin would be negligible.

In man the fate of injected proteins is similar to that in animals

(Madsen 1936), but the reported findings indicate a degree of irregularity not apparent in the animal studies. In the case of horse serum antitoxin the half-life reported, or indicated by the published figures, varies between 4 and 12 days, and it also varies appreciably between individuals (Barr & Sachs 1955; Turner *et al.* 1958; Bergentz & Philipson 1958). A phase of rapid, immune elimination may succeed the catabolic phase in man but it does not appear to occur as regularly in man as in experimental animals. Barr and Sachs (1955) observed immune elimination in 7 of 26 soldiers given antitoxin, and Suri and Rubbo (1961) in only 5 of 30 patients—some of whom had a history of previous antitoxin injection. Cooke and Jones (1943) observed that horse antitoxin, given in large doses therapeutically, can remain circulating for as long as 70 days; it is possible that such prolonged circulation may represent some form of immunological tolerance. The irregularity with which immune elimination occurs is reflected in the findings of Reisman and his colleagues (1961*a*) that antibodies against injected horse serum develop in only a proportion of patients. Of 71 persons given horse antitoxin, 15 developed serum sickness, and each of these had an appreciable titre of pre-existing anti-horse serum antibodies, and each produced a rise in titre in response to the injection. The 56 remaining patients either had no pre-existing antibody or only low titres. Of these 56 only 12 developed antibody in response to the injected horse serum.

As in animals, immune elimination may occur unexpectedly soon after the injection of serum in patients who have received antitoxin previously, and it can also occur immediately if circulating antibody against horse serum is present at the time of injection (see Godfrey *et al.* 1960). On the other hand, a history of having had serum is not necessarily a reliable guide to the likelihood of rapid elimination since Suri and Rubbo (1961) found that the proportion of patients who showed early elimination of antitoxin was no different in those with and without a history of having had serum previously.

*In summary*, the half-life of horse serum antitoxin in man is normally about 7 days, but the elimination rate from the circulation may be rapidly accelerated owing to an immune response, although this by no means always occurs. Early elimination may be expected in perhaps 10 to 25 per cent of patients, although the proportion may be lower in the developing countries where fewer persons will have had previous injections of horse serum. The immune elimination may occur particularly early in a proportion of those who have had horse serum previously, and may start immediately in those already possessing circulating antibodies against the foreign horse proteins. Hypersensitivity reactions such as anaphylaxis or serum sickness may accompany the immune elimination.

*The dose of antitoxin* which should be given for prophylaxis is difficult to decide. There is reluctance to give a large dose on the grounds that this may be more liable to sensitize the patient. On the other hand a small dose may not circulate in sufficient concentration and for long enough to give reliable protection. The dose of horse antitoxin recommended by different authors has indeed varied widely—from 1500 to 10,000 units and even more. In World War I the British Army increased the dose from the 500 units used at first to 1500 units and, although no advantage could be shown for the larger amount, 1500 units has been the most commonly used dose in Great Britain and elsewhere since that time.

When 1500 units of horse antitoxin are given intramuscularly in adults the available evidence (see Suri & Rubbo 1961; Rubinstein 1962; McComb & Dwyer 1963) indicates that the serum concentration does not reach a peak until about 2 days after injection, when a concentration of between 0·2 and 0·5 units per ml may be expected. The level then falls steadily and, in the absence of an immune elimination phase, can be expected to be between 0·05 and 0·1 unit per ml at about 10 or 14 days and between 0·01 and 0·05 unit at 3 weeks. Protection against tetanus should thus be present for about 3 weeks after the usual 1500 unit dose, provided immune elimination dose not occur.

In a proportion of wounded persons antitoxin prophylaxis can be expected to fail. Antitoxin may be given too late, i.e. after a dangerous dose of toxin has been taken up into the central nervous system. It may also be expected to fail if toxin is produced in very large amounts in a severe infection. Since it is necessary for antitoxin to circulate until toxin production has ceased, antitoxin prophylaxis may also fail when early immune elimination of the horse serum occurs and, in the absence of this, if tetanus bacilli continue to multiply in a lesion for a long period, i.e. over 3 weeks. It is not therefore surprising that very many records exist of patients who have developed tetanus in spite of antitoxin injections—the 'tetanus post-sérique' of the French authors. Bianchi (1962), for example, collected reports of 5057 such cases occurring between 1912 and

1960, and in a number of reported series of cases a significant proportion of the patients had had antitoxin promptly at the time of injury, e.g. 6 of 33 patients reported by Cox *et al.* (1963). Figures such as these have been quoted to support the suggestion that 1500 units of antitoxin is insufficient for prophylaxis, and that larger doses should be used routinely, e.g. 50 units per kg body weight, or perhaps 6000 units for all injured persons.

An increase in the dose of antitoxin to 6000 units should give a peak serum antitoxin concentration about 4 times higher than after the usual 1500 unit dose (i.e. about 1·6 units per ml), and the serum level should remain above 0·01 unit for perhaps 5 weeks instead of 3 weeks. Although the larger dose might therefore be expected to prevent tetanus in an additional number of patients, there are a number of arguments against its routine use. In the first place only a small number of additional patients would be protected by the larger dose, i.e. those in whom a four-fold increase in the circulating antitoxin concentration makes the difference between prophylactic failure and success, together with those in whom the extra 14 days protection does so. Thus, even where tetanus is common, less than 1 in 7000 patients given 1500 units of antitoxin for an injury develop the disease. Even if 6000 units was four times better, which seems unlikely, the incidence would be reduced from say 1 : 7000 to 1 : 28,000 so that at best only 3 : 28,000 patients would benefit. This added protective effect would be acceptable if the injection of horse antitoxin were harmless, but it is probable that the increased dose of antigen would give rise to more hypersensitivity reactions and to a greater likelihood of immune elimination—in which case protection would not last for the expected 4–5 weeks. Furthermore, although the evidence that 1500 units is an effective prophylactic dose is admittedly incomplete, there is no good evidence that a bigger dose is better. *In view of these considerations we recommend that* 1500 *units, given s.c. or i.m. is an acceptable prophylactic dose where horse serum must be used.* In patients whose wound is still considered to be a potential source of tetanus toxin 2–3 weeks after a first injection of 1500 units of antitoxin, further protection may be provided by a second dose of 1500 units.

*The effectiveness of passive heterologous antitoxin* is frequently doubted. As mentioned above, an appreciable proportion of the tetanus patients seen in many hospitals have had antitoxin and there are numerous records of its having failed to prevent the disease.

These failures cannot be regarded as sufficient evidence to condemn passive protection. It is only to be expected that in countries where injured persons are routinely given antitoxin, tetanus cases will consist largely of a mixture of those who had very trivial injuries and did not bother to seek medical care, together with patients in whom the prophylactic measures have failed. Nevertheless, the evidence that horse antitoxin does prevent tetanus when given to wounded persons is, unfortunately, inconclusive; it can be summarized as follows:

1 Heterologous antitoxin is able to prevent the development of tetanus in experimentally infected animals.

2 Bruce's (1920) analysis of 1458 cases of tetanus among 1,242,000 wounded soldiers returned to Great Britain from France in World War I presents evidence that antitoxin is effective and has often been quoted. However, the main findings deserve some consideration.

(*a*) Bruce showed that after prophylactic antitoxin was made available in large quantities in France, so that all wounded soldiers could receive 500 units (in terms of the international unit of today), the incidence of tetanus fell from 9 per thousand wounded in September 1914 to 1·4 per thousand in December 1914. Unfortunately, this fall cannot be taken as proof that antitoxin was the cause—other factors, such as the increasing efficiency of the field surgical care, or alterations in the character of the battle—could have been responsible. A fall of similar magnitude (6·5-fold) occurred at other times during the war when no change in the use of antitoxin was made, e.g. from 2·3 cases per thousand wounded in April 1915, to 0·2 cases per thousand in June 1915 (an 11-fold reduction).

(*b*) The use of antitoxin appeared to cause a prolongation of the average incubation period from 12 days in 1914 to 50 days in 1917. Since these figures are derived from wounded patients returned to Great Britain, it is possible that patients with a shorter incubation period may not have reached the country. The figures could therefore reflect the possibility that later on in the war wounded soldiers remained in France for a longer time before being returned to Britain. On the other hand, their validity is supported by Bruce's observation that the average incubation period was 11 days in tetanus patients who had not been given antitoxin and 45 days in those who had had antitoxin. This prolongation of the incubation period suggests that toxin can be prevented from reaching the central nervous system whilst passive antitoxin remains circulating—a period of about 2 weeks after a dose of 500 units (Fildes 1929). It does remain possible, however, that treatment of protected and unprotected patients may have differed in other respects such as the standard of surgical care, and this could influence the incubation period.

(*c*) The crude fatality rate from tetanus in patients who had had prophylactic antitoxin was 22·5 per cent, compared with 53·5 per cent among patients either not given antitoxin or in whom its injection was not recorded. Again, it might be argued that the treatment given to patients who failed to receive their antitoxin might have differed in other ways that could account for these findings.

(*d*) During the war the proportion of patients with only local tetanus increased from 1 : 99 in 1914 to 1 : 3·2 in 1917. This is attributed to the ability of passive antitoxin to neutralize toxin travelling to the central nervous system *via* the blood-stream more easily than toxin spreading into nerves in the vicinity of the infected area. Thus pure local tetanus can be produced experimentally by injecting toxin intramuscularly into protected rabbits. However, this evidence is not beyond criticism because, as Bruce pointed out, improved diagnosis might have accounted in part for the increased proportion of local tetanus.

It appears that the evidence from World War I does not fully meet the criteria considered necessary nowadays to establish the effectiveness of treatment, but taken together the evidence is undoubtedly very suggestive that antitoxin is of value in prophylaxis.

3 Bazy (1914) described 200 wounded soldiers, of whom 100 were not given antitoxin for reasons which he did not state. Eighteen cases of tetanus developed in the unprotected group and only one in the protected group—and that occurred on the day after the antitoxin was given. Although the details given are too few for this report to be accepted as a controlled trial, the results again suggest that antitoxin is effective.

4 The fall in the incidence of tetanus following blank-cartridge injuries in the annual independence celebrations in the U.S.A., from 1 in 4·27 to virtually none over a period of about 12 years at the beginning of this century, has been attributed to the introduction of antitoxin prophylaxis, but it is clearly impossible to exclude other factors operating over this period.

5 The incidence of tetanus in the contesting armies in the Polish campaign of 1939 was 0·036 per cent in the German wounded, in whom antitoxin was freely used, and 0·66 per cent in the Polish wounded for whom supplies of antitoxin were limited. The difference in incidence may have been due to the use of antitoxin, but numerous other factors must have differed in the prepared German and unprepared Polish forces.

The evidence given above is very suggestive that prophylaxis with horse serum antitoxin does have a valuable effect in man, as indeed would be expected from a knowledge of the pathological process. However, since no properly controlled field study has been made, the true value of antitoxin cannot finally be decided. In summary, therefore, it is probable that horse antitoxin does have a prophylactic effect in man but, in the authors' opinion, there is little justification for increasing the routine prophylactic dose above 1500 units.

Passive immunization has a number of disadvantages apart from the fact that it sometimes fails to prevent tetanus. Like any passive measure, it cannot prevent tetanus in patients who do not come for medical care because their injury is minor or unnoticed—such patients can be protected only by active immunization. In addition, there are two disadvantages implicit in the use of heterologous serum, namely, immune elimination and hypersensitivity reactions. Immune elimination has already been discussed (p. 46).

*Hypersensitivity reactions* to injected horse serum may take the form of a local reaction at the injection site, consisting of varying degrees of erythema, swelling, irritation and pain; they can be severe, and occasionally the swelling involves the whole limb. Local reactions may develop within 2 days of injection or be delayed for about 5 to 10 days. Generalized serum sickness may also occur, usually about 10 to 14 days after injection, but sometimes in the accelerated form within a few days of giving the serum. Acute anaphylaxis, developing immediately or within an hour of the injection, is the hypersensitivity reaction which is most feared because, although rare, it can be fatal—anaphylaxis has been estimated to cause death in about one in every 200,000 recipients of horse serum (Laurent & Parish 1952). Neuritis may occur in association with serum sickness and can leave permanent weaknesses and muscular atrophy (Bardenwerper 1962). The overall incidence of reactions has been variously estimated at from 5 to as much as 50 per cent, some of this variation being attributable to differences in the criteria accepted as indicating a reaction, and in the thoroughness of follow-up. Hypersensitivity may be commoner in the developed countries than in the developing countries, because a greater proportion of their populations has had injections of horse serum in the past.

Allergic reactions are dependent on the development by the patient of an immunological response against the injected horse serum proteins, and it is probable that both circulating antibodies and delayed-type (or cell-mediated) hypersensitivity against the foreign proteins can be involved. It is therefore to be expected that hypersensitivity reactions are more likely to occur in patients who have received antitoxin previously, because they may already have developed an immunological reaction against horse serum as a result of the previous injection. Thus the chance of developing serum sickness has been related to the titre of horse serum antibodies already present at the time of injection (Reisman *et al.* 1961*a*). Moynihan (1955) investigated 7580 patients and recorded an incidence of serum reactions of 2·5 per cent. In 909 of the patients who were believed to have had serum previously, the incidence of reactions was 5·7 per cent. Binns (1961) found the incidence of local and general reactions to be 10·5 per cent after reinjection, compared with 8·7 per cent after first injection. These recent reports record a surprisingly small increase in the frequency with which reactions follow re-injection of refined horse serum—possibly because patients often do not know whether or not they have had horse serum previously.

A local reaction at the site of an injection of antitoxin may sometimes be seen a number of hours before the development of a generaized reaction (Binns 1961). This local response may be due to the interaction of serum remaining at the injection site and antibody which has developed against it but, whatever the cause, it is an indication for starting antihistamine therapy with the aim of preventing or attenuating the generalized illness.

*A test for hypersensitivity* should always be made before horse serum is injected, and if hypersensitivity is detected horse serum antitoxin should not be given for prophylaxis. This recommendation is justified because:

1 In patients who are demonstrably hypersensitive it is unwise to risk the severe reaction that may follow the full dose of antitoxin.

2 A reaction to the test dose implies the presence of antibodies

against horse serum which may well cause immediate or accelerated immune elimination of the injected serum.

Thus injection of serum into a hypersensitive patient is dangerous and may also be useless. If it possible to desensitize the patient by injecting first a minute dose of the antitoxin, followed at intervals by further doses which are slowly increased in size, provided no adverse response occurs. This process is difficult to justify for prophylaxis because the patient will probably quickly produce fresh antibody which will eliminate the horse serum and rapidly terminate its effect and may, at the same time, produce hypersensitivity reactions.

*In the case of a patient with clinical tetanus* who is hypersensitive to horse serum (i.e. has a history of previous reactions to horse serum, or gives a general reaction to the trial dose (*vide infra*)) the therapeutic effect of a short period of circulation of antitoxin may be thought to justify the desensitizing procedure, but in view of the probably limited therapeutic effect of an injection of antitoxin (p. 104) it would be equally justifiable to withhold horse serum in such patients. In many countries it should be possible to provide human antitoxin for this small group of patients.

The type of test for hypersensitivity to horse serum which should be used cannot be decided with certainty, since there is insufficient evidence available. Parish and his colleagues (Laurent & Parish 1952; Parish & Cannon 1961) claim that both intradermal and conjunctival tests are unreliable because they give both false-positive and false-negative results. They believe that the test dose should be used as an attempt to recognize patients who run a risk of developing anaphylaxis, and recommend that the test should consist of a small 'trial' dose of serum given subcutaneously; the patient is then observed for not less than half an hour for evidence of a generalized reaction, and they suggest that local reactions to the trial dose should be ignored. The use of a subcutaneous trial dose as Parish recommends seems a very reasonable procedure, but a local reaction to a trial dose of antitoxin presumably does indicate the presence of antibodies against some component of the injected serum which, even if insufficient to produce anaphylaxis, might nevertheless be associated with severe local reactions or the development of serum sickness when the full dose is given. Although Cox *et al.* (1963) found no association between a local reaction to the trial dose and later reactions to the whole dose, Binns (1961) found that in patients who developed a local reaction within one hour of receiving a trial dose of antitoxin, the incidence of later generalized reactions was four times greater than in patients who had had no local reaction. Consequently the development of a local reaction to a trial dose of horse serum can sometimes be a warning that the patient has an increased liability to respond unfavourably to horse serum even though both false-positive and false-negative results undoubtedly occur. The principle of the trial dose is valuable because acute anaphylaxis is certainly the reaction to be most feared, but *we believe that local as well as general reactions should be regarded as a contra-indication to the injection of horse serum for tetanus prophylaxis.* In the more urgent case of the patient requiring treatment of clinical tetanus, a local reaction to the trial dose would not suffice to justify withholding horse antitoxin treatment, but in such cases the serum should be given cautiously.

The amount of antitoxin to be given as a trial dose in testing for hypersensitivity is debatable. If the dose is too small it is possible that some hypersensitive patients may fail to react and, if too large, the test itself may provoke a severe, and even fatal, reaction. A dose of 0·05 ml (i.e. 75 units) of the ordinary pepsin-refined antitoxin (e.g. Tet/Ser, B.P.), injected subcutaneously, is a reasonable compromise. It must be pointed out that even this small dose is not completely safe; fatal anaphylaxis has occurred after the injection of 0·01 ml of horse antitoxin (Buff 1960). The patient should be observed for at least half an hour after receiving the trial dose and, if no reaction has then developed, the remainder of the dose may be given. Whenever antitoxin is given—whether as a small trial dose or as a full prophylactic or therapeutic dose—adrenaline 1/1000 (Adrenaline Injection B.P.) should be available for immediate use in case acute anaphylaxis develops.

*In patients with a history of any allergy*, horse serum antitoxin should be given with even more than usual caution, owing to the greater risk of provoking a reaction. A history of allergy should always be carefully enquired for and if elicited should lead to a reconsideration of the need to inject the foreign protein. When it is, nevertheless, decided to give antitoxin, the usual trial dose should be preceded by a smaller trial dose—0·05 ml of a 1/10 dilution of the antitoxin. If no reaction has developed after half an hour the usual test dose of 0·05 ml of undiluted antitoxin must then be given before proceeding to inject the full dose.

*The injection of heterologous serum into patients who have had a previous injection* should clearly be avoided whenever possible. The patient who is given horse antitoxin is left at a therapeutically-induced disadvantage compared to his fellows in that, should he be given a subsequent injection of heterologous serum, he has a greater likelihood of developing a hypersensitivity reaction and of eliminating the antiserum with undue rapidity. In such patients treatment with horse serum may be both dangerous and useless. It should therefore be the responsibility of the doctor who gives horse serum to ensure that the therapeutic disadvantage is overcome, so that his patient will not need horse serum again. This can be done by actively immunizing the patient against those diseases for which passive horse serum may be used, i.e. for practical purposes, tetanus and perhaps diphtheria in countries where the disease is common. Active immunization against tetanus can most conveniently be initiated at the time when the horse serum is given, and it is advocated that for routine purposes passive immunization with horse serum for tetanus prophylaxis should always be accompanied by a simultaneous injection of adsorbed tetanus toxoid (see p. 71).

It does not seem justifiable to recommend that a history of previously having had horse serum is a complete contraindication to its reinjection since second injections often produce no ill-effects (e.g. Moynihan 1955), and often provide circulating antitoxin for the usual time (Suri & Rubbo 1961). The policy we recommend is that horse serum should be given to such patients only if there is a clear indication to do so, such as a severe, dirty wound, or a patient with clinical tetanus.

*Human anti-tetanus immunoglobulin* has become available in recent years in a number of European countries and in North America and has been the subject of a number of studies (e.g. Rubbo & Suri 1962; Rubinstein 1962; McComb & Dwyer 1963). Human antitoxin is given in the form of the gamma-globulin fraction, rather than as whole serum, because when properly prepared this fraction is free from the risk of transmitting serum hepatitis and because the antibodies from a large amount of serum can be injected in a conveniently small volume. Although human gamma-immunoglobulins do possess allotypic antigens and corresponding antibodies have been found in the serum of treated patients, there seems little doubt that for practical purposes human anti-tetanus immunoglobulin can be regarded as non-antigenic in man. Consequently human antitoxin is not liable to immune elimination, so that, unlike heterologous horse antitoxin, its period of passive protection will not be unexpectedly shortened. Moreover, it is not liable to provoke hypersensitivity reactions and is therefore safe when given intramuscularly or subcutaneously.

The preparations at present in use occasionally give rise to adverse reactions when injected intravenously—probably caused by aggregated gamma-globulin molecules. The reactions may take the form of discomfort, flushing of the face, or circulatory collapse with loss of consciousness. The risk of causing collapse is clearly a drawback to the use of human anti-tetanus immunoglobulin for treatment, when intravenous injection is preferable in order to achieve a high concentration of antitoxin in the blood as rapidly as possible.

Homologous antitoxin has the additional advantage of possessing a long half-life, variously reported to be from 20 to 43 days, so that a small dose of antitoxin will circulate for a prolonged period. Apart from the advantages already referred to there have been suggestions that homologous antitoxin is more effective, unit for unit, than heterologous antitoxin. However, a recent comparative study in animals failed to support this view (Smith 1967), so that for *treatment* of tetanus the dose of homologous antitoxin should be the same as that of heterologous horse serum antitoxin. For *prophylaxis* small doses can be employed because, owing to its long half-life, a dose of only 250 units will provide a serum antitoxin concentration of more than 0·01 unit per ml for about four weeks. With heterologous antitoxin, on the other hand, a large dose has to be given to ensure that adequate blood levels are still present two or three weeks later.

The dose of human antitoxin that should be used for prophylaxis has received much discussion. Because the rate of elimination is slow and has no immune phase, it is possible to choose a dose that will provide, within reasonable limits, a serum antitoxin concentration above any desired minimum, for any required period of time. The amount injected need not be restricted on the grounds of safety or fear of sensitization. It would, for example, be possible to use a dose which provided a serum antitoxin concentration serum over 0·1 units for more than 6 weeks. However, as might be expected, it is necessary to limit dosage on grounds of supply, so that most authors have been concerned to estimate the smallest dose that can be considered protective. McComb (1964) has produced convincing arguments that the protective dose of human antitoxin can be as low as 250 units for adults and has supported his view by drawing on the wide experience that has been obtained in preventing tetanus in horses, for which homologous equine antitoxin has long been used. In man the 250-unit dose of human antitoxin has now been widely accepted (*Lancet* 1966), and after intramuscular injection into adults this produces a serum concentration of approximately 0·025 unit per ml at 2 days; 4 weeks later the concentration is still between 0·01 and 0·025 unit per ml.

There is some evidence that the peak serum concentration of human antitoxin occurs later in man after intramuscular injection, and the peak attained is apparently a little higher, than is the case with horse antitoxin. Rubinstein (1962) found the highest antitoxin level at 5 days after injection of human antitoxin and 2 days after injection of horse antitoxin. These observations may be accounted for by a slower absorption of homologous protein from the injection site, but a more important factor is probably the faster catabolism of the horse globulin, so that an appreciable amount has already been eliminated by the fifth day.

There seems little doubt that an injection of human antitoxin is the treatment of choice for non-immune patients who require prophylaxis in addition to that provided by surgical débridement, even though there is no field evidence of its effectiveness. Since Nocard's work the evidence that homologous antitoxin is highly effective in horses has steadily accumulated, and there is little reason to doubt that homologous antitoxin is equally effective in man.

The major difficulty in recommending the widespread use of human antitoxin is that of supply. To achieve adequate yields by the methods at present in use, the serum to be fractionated must be obtained from immunized volunteers who have recently received a booster dose of tetanus toxoid. At about 10 days after boosting, the serum antitoxin concentration may be between 2 and 30 units per ml, depending on the individual patient and on other factors, including the type of vaccine used; highest yields are obtained with vaccines containing immunological adjuvants, such as aluminium hydroxide. Fractionation of 1 litre of serum containing 20 units per ml may be expected to yield about 50 ml of 16 per cent gamma-globulin solution containing 300 units of antitoxin per ml (assuming an 80 per cent recovery and a 15-fold concentration in antibody content). Thus a donation from one patient (say 350 ml of serum) may provide a 250-unit prophylactic dose for perhaps 22 patients. To replace the extremely large amounts of horse serum antitoxin which are used in the world it is clear that volunteer donors would be required in very large numbers. However, the widespread use of active immunization could result in the demand for passive protection becoming small enough to be met without great difficulty, and in some countries, e.g. U.S.A., Holland, Switzerland, human antitoxin is now widely available.

*Bovine and ovine antitoxins* have also been used for prophylaxis and treatment and, although they have no therapeutic advantage over horse antitoxin, there is some slight evidence that purified bovine antitoxin may be less liable to provoke hypersensitivity reactions in man than purified horse antitoxin. Of greater interest is the possibility that bovine or ovine antitoxin could be used with safety in patients who are hypersensitive to horse serum. This procedure cannot be recommended wholeheartedly because there are antigenic relationships between the gamma–globulins of different animal species, and antibodies against equine gamma-globulin are likely to show some reactivity with bovine gamma-globulin (Regamey 1953; Reisman *et al.* 1961*b*). Consequently, a proportion of patients hypersensitive to horse serum may be expected to develop reactions if injected with bovine antitoxin and they may also rapidly eliminate the antitoxin from the circulation. However, when Trinca and Reid (1967) gave bovine antitoxin to 69 wounded persons, 25 of whom had previously reacted to horse serum, only 3 patients had reactions to the bovine serum and these were only minor and local. Although there is a possibility that bovine antitoxin may be safe for patients sensitive to horse serum, there is no doubt that an injection of human gamma-globulin antitoxin is greatly to be preferred. If human antitoxin is not available and it is considered essential to provide passive protection for a patient hypersensitive to horse serum, another heterologous antiserum should not be given unless a test dose has provoked no reaction.

# 7
# PREVENTION OF TETANUS 3

## *Active immunization*

Man can be immunized effectively against tetanus by spaced injections of tetanus formol toxoid. Although no controlled trial has been conducted, the efficacy of active immunization is evident not only from experiments in animals but also from the extremely low incidence of tetanus in the immunized British and American forces in World War II. Among 2½ million wounded American soldiers only 12 developed tetanus; and some of these may not have had all their toxoid injections (Long & Sartwell 1947). Active immunization is not only highly effective but it is also the only means whereby tetanus following minor unnoticed injuries can be prevented.

*Tetanus toxoid* is produced from the culture filtrate of a toxogenic strain of *Clostridium tetani*. The filtrate is purified and treated with formaldehyde long enough to detoxify the toxin without significantly impairing its antigenicity. The resulting 'formol toxoid' (or plain toxoid, as it may be called) is tested in animals to ensure its immunizing potency and freedom from toxicity; it can then be used for immunization in man (e.g. Tet/Vac,B.P.).

*The concentration of toxoid* in a vaccine is often expressed in Lf units, which are a measure of its ability to combine and visibly flocculate with Standard tetanus antitoxin; thus 1 Lf can be thought of as the amount of toxoid which is equivalent to one unit of antitoxin. An immunizing dose of tetanus toxoid may, for example, contain 20 Lf in a volume of 0·5 ml. Although the Lf value bears some relationship to the immunizing potency of a vaccine, this is not necessarily the case because there are undoubtedly other factors, many of which are not understood, that effect the potency of vaccine.

Although tetanus toxoid is a good antigen, much of the vaccine produced today incorporates an immunological adjuvant, such as an aluminium salt, to increase its immunizing potency (e.g. Tet/Vac

PTAH,B.P.). Aluminium adjuvants probably act by increasing the local inflammatory response to the injected antigen, which can lead to appreciable local antibody formation, and also a depot of antigen is formed from which the toxoid is slowly released over a prolonged period. It is also probable that small depots are formed elsewhere in the body as a result of small amounts of the vaccine escaping from the site of injection. Tetanus formol toxoid adsorbed on to aluminium hydroxide or aluminium phosphate has been shown to stimulate antitoxin formation more quickly than when given without an adjuvant, to stimulate a higher serum antitoxin concentration, and to produce a longer lasting immunity (see, for example, Gottlieb *et al.* 1964). In addition, aluminium adjuvant toxoid has been shown to be effective when given in a separate injection but at the same time as passive antitoxin immunization (see p. 71), whereas doubt exists about the use of plain toxoid in these circumstances (Smith 1964). Adsorbed toxoid has the possible disadvantage that it may cause more local reactions than plain formol toxoid owing to the irritant effect of the aluminium adjuvant, but when given by deep intramuscular injection the evidence so far available indicates that reactions are not significantly more frequent than following plain toxoid injections (White & Ungar 1967). In view of the advantages possessed by the adsorbed toxoid, the authors consider that for routine use it is the preparation of choice. It has been argued that plain toxoid should be given when a booster effect is required in previously immunized persons because there is some evidence that, in contrast to the findings in primary immunization, it induces a detectable rise in the serum antitoxin concentration sooner than adsorbed toxoid (Miller *et al.* 1949). However, in the study concerned the toxoids used may not have been genuinely comparable and, more recently, Trinca (1965) was unable to detect any difference in the rate of the booster response to the two types of toxoid; adsorbed toxoid is therefore recommended for all patients.

Pertussis vaccine acts as an immunological adjuvant, probably by virtue of its endotoxin content, and in the combined vaccines used for immunization of children the pertussis component enhances the response to the other antigens—including the tetanus toxoid. Aluminium adjuvants are therefore not always used in vaccines containing pertussis.

Oil adjuvants are currently receiving much study, with the particular aim of producing a vaccine able to stimulate immunity with a single injection, and for this purpose highly concentrated toxoids are also being studied. Mineral and vegetable oils can act as powerful immunological adjuvants. Their action is probably attributable to local inflammation, together with prolonged retention and slow release of antigen, but a degree of general stimulation of antibody-forming tissues may also be involved. A 'single-dose' vaccine would be particularly valuable in the developing countries for the immunization of pregnant women in order to prevent *tetanus neonatorum* and puerperal tetanus. The various oils that have been employed as adjuvants are often very effective in enhancing the antibody response, but are often unacceptably irritant, and preparations suitable for general use are not yet available.

*The route of injection* which most workers prefer is deep intramuscular; this route is particularly important with adsorbed toxoids that are expected to produce a small granuloma, which may be uncomfortable and obvious if the injection is given superficially. The intradermal route is not advised for routine use because there is evidence that it gives rise to a high incidence of reactions (White & Ungar 1967), but this route is used for vaccines in which tetanus is combined with typhoid and paratyphoid antigens (Barr *et al.* 1959); typhoid vaccine given in a suitable dose intradermally provokes fewer generalized reactions than when given by deeper injection.

A large dose of tetanus toxoid, when injected into an animal, can specifically protect the animal against a lethal amount of toxin injected a few hours afterwards—long before antitoxin can be produced. This 'specific precocious protective action' is attributed to the toxoid competing with toxin for its receptor site in nervous tissue. The amount of toxoid that must be given in order to protect in this way is large, and the phenomenon is not thought to be of practical prophylactic value in man (Davies & Wright 1955).

*The schedule of toxoid injections* that has been recommended by different workers varies considerably, but all follow certain principles, and the schedule used in Britain can be used as an example. The basic immunizing course consists of three injections suitably spaced. The first dose stimulates a primary antibody response, the most important effect of which is a conditioning of the antibody-forming tissues of the host so that, when a second injection of toxoid is given, a 'secondary antibody response' occurs—characterized by the speedy production of antitoxin in substantial quantities. The second injection must therefore be delayed until the state of 'secondary responsiveness' has developed; there is evidence that such responsiveness can be expected 3 weeks after the first injection but that its degree increases if the interval is lengthened to 6 or 9 weeks. In practice it is convenient to employ a short interval, and 4 or 6 weeks is widely recommended. The third injection, which is sometimes called the 'reinforcing dose' (Edsall 1967), is given 6 to 12 months after the second, and aims at stimulating an even greater response to the toxoid, i.e. a response characterized by the production of a high concentration of circulating antitoxin leading to an immunity which can last for as long as 20 years. It should be emphasized that the basic immunization course consists of all three of the spaced injections. This course is sometimes referred to as the primary immunization course, which is a little confusing because immunologists may refer to the *first* injection as the primary immunization, stimulating as it does a primary antibody response. We therefore prefer that the course of injections is termed the basic immunizing course.

In infants under 6 months immunized with multiple antigens, for example diphtheria-tetanus-pertussis vaccine, it is sometimes advised to give three injections at 4-week intervals, followed by a fourth injection 6 to 12 months later. The extra initial injection is given to ensure that the response will be adequate even though the young infant may not be immunologically mature (Evans & Smith 1963).

Active immunization of women, either during pregnancy or up to 5 years previously, with two injections of adsorbed toxoid at not less than 1 month's interval, has been shown to be highly effective in preventing *tetanus neonatorum* by means of the passive transfer of the maternal antitoxin to the baby (MacLennan *et al.* 1965; Newell *et al.* 1966).

It should be noted that an attack of tetanus does not confer immunity to the disease, probably because the lethal dose of toxin is so very small that a person recovering from the disease is unlikely to have had sufficient toxin in his tissues to act as an immunizing dose.

*Booster injections of toxoid* are those that are given after the basic course in order to enhance and prolong the immunity which otherwise might wane and disappear. The frequency with which they should be given, indeed whether they are required at all, is a controversial matter. Even quite recently the use of 3- or 5-yearly toxoid injections was recommended (e.g. Edsall 1959), but evidence has accumulated that immunity lasts for many years after a properly spaced basic course of injections of adsorbed toxoid (e.g. Scheibel *et al.* 1966; Rubbo 1966). Consequently, recent recommendations have varied between requiring booster doses to be given every 10 years to the suggestion that the basic course induces a life-long immunity.

From the available evidence it is probable that antitoxin will circulate in the majority of individuals for 10 years after the basic immunization course with adsorbed toxoid, and that a good response to a booster injection can be expected up to this time. It may well be that immunity lasts much longer than 10 years, but *we recommend that a booster dose should be given at 10 years after primary immunization except where there is good evidence that the available vaccines do provide immunity of a longer duration.* In Britain at the present time, for example, the evidence is not yet strong enough to recommend delaying the booster injection for more than 10 years after the basic immunization course. After a booster of adsorbed toxoid has been given at 10 years, it seems likely that lifelong immunity will result, although this cannot be regarded as proven. In patients immunized with plain toxoid, on the other hand (up to about 1964 only plain toxoid was used in Britain), immunity may not be so long-lasting (White *et al.* 1967) and a booster at 5 years after the primary course is advisable, together with a second booster about 10 years later, immunity will then probably be lifelong.

For children who have been immunized in infancy a booster should be given at the age of about 5 years, preferably in the form of a combined diphtheria and tetanus vaccine, as recommended by the Ministry of Health (1963). This procedure should ensure adequate immunity in adolescence and early adult life when the risk of wounding is possibly greater. Recent work in USA however suggests that four spaced injections of absorbed toxoid in infancy gives immunity for 12 years (Peebles *et al.* 1969). Until more is known about the duration of immunity in children immunized in this way, it is advisable to give a further booster injection of adsorbed tetanus toxoid at around 16 years of age; immunity will then probably be lifelong. For those in whom the occupational risk of tetanus is high, for example farm workers and soldiers, 10-yearly boosting is probably desirable.

*A booster injection of toxoid at the time of injury* is commonly given. In persons never previously immunized, the aim is to grasp the opportunity to initiate active immunization; the injection has no immediate prophylactic effect, but serves as the first dose of the basic immunization course. In actively immunized patients the injection is given to stimulate a rise in the serum antitoxin concentration at a time when this might be needed and, in addition, to enhance and prolong the patient's immunity. This practice was adopted by the U.S. Army in World War II, but not by the British forces. The U.S. experience showed that tetanus is so rare in actively immunized patients who receive a booster dose at the time of injury that it can now be considered as a standard procedure. However, an injection of toxoid is not necessarily protective in all actively immunized patients who are wounded, and may be undesirable in others. Two special cases must be considered—those patients who were last immunized many years previously and, secondly, the recently immunized.

After active immunization the serum antitoxin content slowly declines with the passage of time (e.g. see Gottlieb *et al.* 1964, 1967), and it is probable that the speed with which fresh antitoxin appears in the blood in response to a booster injection also decreases. Consequently, the patient immunized many years previously may not only have little or no circulating antitoxin, but also may respond to the toxoid given at the time of injury too slowly, i.e. tetanus may develop before a protective amount of antitoxin appears in the serum. As discussed above, it is probable that an adequate response can be expected up to 10 years after proper basic immunization, but there is limited evidence concerning periods of time beyond 10 years. Consequently, when more than 10 years have elapsed since basic immunization, the possibility must be borne in mind that a toxoid booster may not be adequate for prophylaxis. In the patient who has had a booster dose of toxoid in addition to the basic immunization course, it is likely that immunity will be lifelong, and for such persons a booster at the time of injury will be fully adequate for prophylaxis although, again, this cannot be regarded as proven.

The second type of case that must be considered is the recently immunized patient who is injured. If it was recommended that a booster should be given as a matter of routine when an injury occurs, some persons, such as industrial workers, could be injected every few months or so whenever they receive a minor wound. Such a practice is unnecessary because the recently immunized will have a high concentration of antitoxin in the circulation and should not require the additional protection given by a booster. Moreover, it is undesirable to inject patients with an antigen repeatedly, since very little is known about the effect of hyperimmunization—hypersensitivity reactions to tetanus toxoid are certainly more likely to occur when repeated injections are given, and it is possible that other harmful effects such as serum protein abnormalities or impaired immunological responsiveness might result (Peeler *et al.* 1965).

In view of these considerations it seems wise to avoid routinely giving a booster to wounded patients who have recently had a dose of toxoid. At the International Conference on Tetanus held in 1966 in Berne (Report 1967) it was agreed that a booster at injury should be avoided in the 12 months following the injection of a previous booster or the third injection of the basic immunization course. However, in the industrial worker in whom frequent minor injuries occur, this recommendation could result in an annual toxoid booster, and the injection of antigens at even this interval is probably undesirable. In view of the accumulating evidence that in properly immunized persons immunity lasts for many years after the last toxoid injection, it seems reasonable to extend the time limit for patients who have already had one toxoid booster over and above their primary course. It is therefore suggested that a repeat booster is unnecessary within 3 years of a previous booster except in those few cases where the patient has a wound which is regarded as particularly 'tetanus-prone' (p. 39). For the patient with a severe tetanus-prone wound it is reasonable to give a booster even though he has had one in the recent past. Patients are unlikely to receive frequent boosters on this account as severe wounding is not a frequent occurrence, and, in addition, in such cases the surgeon is justified in wanting to ensure that every possible precaution has been taken to prevent tetanus.

A question which must also be considered is the reliability of a booster injection for prophylaxis in injured persons who have had an incomplete course of injections. The immune status between the first and second injections depends in part on the nature of the toxoid employed. In general, when adsorbed toxoid has been given most patients will have over 0·01 units of antitoxin per ml of serum 4 weeks after the first dose, but if plain toxoid is given antitoxin will probably not develop until after the second injection. However, some toxoid preparations have a low potency and not all adsorbed toxoids can be relied upon to produce a response within 4 weeks (Snyder *et al.* 1966).

It is probable that most people will be immune in the interval between the second and third doses of the basic immunization course (Evans 1943) and would not require a booster dose if injured at this time.

There is very little information about the patient who fails to return for the second or third injection of toxoid and this again probably depends on whether an adjuvant toxoid was used. Thus Ericsson (1948) found that 2 to 3 years after immunization with one dose of adsorbed toxoid, which had been given simultaneously with horse antitoxin, 47 per cent of 70 persons possessed circulating antitoxin and 96 per cent had responded to a second injection when examined 2 weeks later. Evans (1965) found circulating antitoxin 19 years after two doses of plain toxoid, and the work of Newell *et al.* (1966) on prevention of *tetanus neonatorum* indicates that two doses of adsorbed toxoid should give protection for at least 5 years.

Conclusions drawn from such sparse information can only be tentative, but probably it is wisest to consider that patients who have had only one injection of toxoid have not had an adequate antigenic stimulus; therefore a second injection given at the time of wounding cannot be relied on for protection. In those who have had two toxoid injections it is likely that for some time afterwards a booster injection will stimulate a rapid antitoxin response and provide adequate prophylaxis, but the time limit for which a booster can be considered reliable must be decided to some extent arbitrarily. In view of the findings of Newell and his colleagues, boosting at the time of wounding must be considered reliable for up to 5 years after two doses of adsorbed toxoid, but since there is little information about immunity after this interval a 5-year limit is suggested.

Recommendations concerning the use of toxoid in actively immunized persons who are wounded can be summarized as follows:

Actively-immunized patients who receive a wound, other than one that is clean, superficial and easily cleaned, should be given an injection of toxoid on wounding except:

1 Within 1 year of the basic immunization course for all patients, provided the wound is not considered particularly 'tetanus-prone'.

2 Within 3 years of a previous booster injection, provided the wound is not considered particularly 'tetanus-prone'.

Additional prophylaxis (i.e. antitoxin or antibotics) should be considered for the following, in whom the toxoid injection may not provide adequate protection:

1 Those who have had only one toxoid injection;

2 Those who have had two injections of toxoid, the last more than 5 years previously;

3 Persons who have had only the basic immunization course more than 10 years previously.

It is regrettable that, although it is possible to suggest clear categories of immunity such as those given above, the various subdivisions are often not particularly helpful in the individual patient who so often does not know what injections he has had, much less when he had them. The treatment necessary for each patient must nevertheless be decided on the basis of what information about his immune status can be discovered and on the considerations discussed above.

The problem of determining the immune status of the individual has received much consideration, and there are a number of possible ways whereby the doctor can be apprised of this information when he is confronted with an injured patient. Thus it is possible to provide the patient with an identity card on which information of medical importance is recorded, including, for example, blood group, hypersensitivities, drugs taken, chronic illness such as diabetes, and also immune status. Such a card has been prepared by the American Medical Association (see Furste *et al.* 1966) but this method suffers from the disadvantage of being unacceptable to those who consider any form of 'identity document' as an infringement on personal liberty and to those who are too lazy or unconcerned to bother. There is also the possibility that the wounded patient will not be carrying his card at the time of injury. The use of a small tattoo mark to record the immune status has a number of advocates, but here again many would consider this unacceptable.

The use of a scheme involving the individual as the carrier of information can be avoided when the whole group from which the patient comes is known to be fully immunized. This is practicable, for example, in the armed forces and in residential schools, but in these circumstances the medical records of the patient are in any case usually readily available at the sick bay. In those parts of the world where immunization schemes can be made compulsory it is possible to immunize such a high proportion of the population that any patient presenting with an injury can be considered immunized. A possibility which is nowadays being considered in a number of countries is that of a central, computerized records system; information about a patient's immune status can then easily be obtained by telephone. In most countries a compromise must be adopted in which records of immunization are kept by general practitioners, casualty departments, schools and other institutions. Patients should also be given a record card at the time of immunization and encouraged to carry it at all times. It is also important to ensure that the patient fully understands the significance of being properly immunized against tetanus and that he knows his immune status.

### *Disadvantages of active immunization*

1 *Slow development of immunity.* When a patient is first immunized against tetanus, the development of immunity is slow; after the first primary injection of adsorbed toxoid it is about 4 weeks before a protective concentration of antitoxin becomes detectable in the blood. Since the incubation period of tetanus is usually less than 3 weeks it is clear that the initiation of active immunization at the time of wounding cannot be relied upon to prevent tetanus developing from that injury.

2 *Failure to prevent tetanus.* It is not really known just how effective immunization with tetanus toxoid is in the general population, because no controlled comparison of the incidence of tetanus in immunized and unimmunized groups has been done. An approach to such a study is the work of Newell and his colleagues (Newell *et al.* 1966) in an area where *tetanus neonatorum* was common. They investigated the incidence of tetanus neonatorum in infants borne by women who were given injections of either adsorbed tetanus toxoid or influenza vaccine during pregnancy, or who had received such injections in the previous 5 years. No cases of tetanus developed in the 341 babies of 517 women given two or more spaced injections of adsorbed toxoid, whereas 27 cases occurred in the 347 babies of 574 women given influenza vaccine. As this work shows, immunization is very effective, but it is also possible that its value is sometimes overestimated.

Thus, tetanus sometimes occurs in persons who have been properly immunized against the disease; the authors have encountered reports of 73 cases, some of which have proved fatal even in patients who had had a booster of toxoid at the time of injury (e.g. Report 1968). At the beginning of this chapter we mentioned the excellent results apparently achieved by active immunization among the American forces in World War II. The incidence of tetanus was 0·44/100,000 compared with 13·4/100,000 in World War I. However, this large difference may in part be accounted for by the better surgical care available in World War II, and, in addition, at the time of wounding the soldiers received a booster injection of toxoid, thus making it difficult to assess the value of the routine basic immunization course: vaccines against most diseases must stand or fall without an additional injection at the time of exposure.

There is no doubt that some persons respond poorly to tetanus toxoid—particularly plain toxoid without adjuvant. White and his colleagues (1967), for example, found that within 4 years of immunization with three spaced injections of plain toxoid, about 10 per cent of adults had less than 0·01 unit of antitoxin per ml of serum. Of persons who had had adsorbed toxoid, all had over 0·01 unit of antitoxin per ml of serum at this time, but a small proportion had only between 0·01 and 0·05 units. It seems likely that, even if active immunization were extended to the whole population, a small number of cases would still occur, presumably in those persons who respond poorly to tetanus toxoid.

3 *Hypersensitivity reactions to toxoid* are not common, but nowadays they are being encountered with increasing frequency, probably because tetanus immunization is now used so widely, particularly in the developed countries. White and Ungar (1966) recorded an incidence of 0·37 per cent for localized and 0·08 per cent for generalized reactions in a factory population in which 20,000 injections of plain toxoid had been given. In 1040 patients, each of whom was seen by a doctor 24 hours after injection so that the follow-up was particularly good, the incidence was found to be 0·5 per cent for local and 0·1 per cent for general reactions. In the case of adsorbed toxoid the incidence was found to be slightly higher—1 per cent and 0·3 per cent for local and general reactions respectively, a difference which was not statistically significant.

Reactions may be localized or generalized, and immediate or delayed in onset, but there has been little work aimed at characterizing the different responses or at determining the type of hypersensitivity involved. The variation in time of onset which may be observed suggests that both reagin-mediated hypersensitivity and delayed-type (cell-mediated) hypersensitivity could be involved, and it is also possible that ordinary circulating or tissue antitoxin is responsible for a proportion of the reactions. Recent evidence suggests that the hypersensitivity is directed against tetanus toxoid itself, rather than against impurities in the vaccine, and that the majority of hypersensitive patients have a good level of immunity (White *et al.* 1968).

The completion of immunization in patients who are hypersensitive to toxoid presents a problem. The development of a reaction implies the occurrence of an immunological response to a component in the vaccine. In the majority of instances this component appears to be the tetanus toxoid itself, and the patients' immunological response also includes circulating antitoxin, i.e. most persons who develop a hypersensitivity reaction to toxoid are immune to tetanus. Nevertheless, with the evidence so far available, it cannot be assumed that all hypersensitive patients are immune and, unless the hypersensitivity is severe, it is advisable to complete the immunization course. There is evidence that in these circumstances immunization can be accomplished safely by injecting a small dose, e.g. 1 Lf of adsorbed toxoid intramuscularly (McComb & Levine 1961; Trinca 1963). Adrenaline 1/1,000 (Adrenaline Injection, B.P.) should be immediately available for treatment of anaphylactic shock whenever toxoid injections are given—as indeed it should be when any material is injected. The prophylactic use of an antihistamine drug is also an advisable precaution.

### *Simultaneous active and passive immunization*

When non-immune persons are treated for a wound it is desirable to initiate, and thereafter to complete, a course of active immunization against tetanus. The adoption of this practice as a matter of routine in casualty departments and by general practitioners would help considerably in the extension of active immunization to as many persons as possible. Such a routine would also be of value in helping to decide the immune status of patients since, if it were known that a person had previously been treated for a wound, it could be inferred that he had had at least one injection of toxoid. Moreover, at the time of injury the patient is most aware of the need to be immunized and is consequently likely to accept, and complete, the immunization course.

When the treatment given to a wounded patient includes passive protection with horse serum antitoxin, the initiation of active immunization is essential. The recipient of horse serum is left at a disadvantage, compared to his fellows, because he has an increased chance of developing a hypersensitivity reaction if he is injected with horse serum again, and is also more likely to eliminate it quickly (see p. 46). This therapeutically-induced disadvantage can largely be overcome by actively immunizing the patient against those diseases in which horse serum may be used for prophylaxis or therapy, i.e. tetanus, diphtheria, gas gangrene, botulism and, possibly, snake bite. In practice, most horse serum is given for tetanus prophylaxis, so that immunization against tetanus should ensure that almost all recipients of horse serum will not need to be given this material again. In countries where diphtheria antitoxin is widely used it is important to ensure that the patient is also properly immunized with diphtheria toxoid. Immunization against gas gangrene, botulism and snake bite is not a practical possibility at present.

There is no doubt that the immune response to tetanus toxoid can be impaired by the simultaneous injection of tetanus antitoxin, and it has often been advocated that the course of active immunization should be delayed for perhaps 6 weeks, when the passive antitoxin will have been completely eliminated from the body. The mechanism by which antibodies impair the immunizing effect of an antigen is not fully understood, but it apparently requires combination of the two to occur *in vivo.* It is possible that the antibody physically blocks antigenic determinants, and also that it effects a rapid elimination of the antigen from the body tissues. In recent years it has become clear that the inhibitory effect of passive antitoxin can be overcome almost entirely with *adsorbed* tetanus toxoid (Eckmann 1963; Smith 1964). Consequently it is recommended that whenever horse serum is given prophylactically, a course of active immunization should be initiated by an injection of adsorbed tetanus toxoid into the opposite arm. The course of immunization should be completed in the usual way.

When passive immunization is practised with human antitoxin, simultaneous active immunization is to be encouraged: even though there is no need to overcome the disadvantages that the recipient of horse serum faces, it is nevertheless desirable to grasp the opportunity to immunize the patient whilst he is aware of the need. Since the dose of human antitoxin given for prophylaxis is only 250 units —one-sixth of the usual 1500-unit dose of horse serum antitoxin— it might be expected that interference with the active response would be negligible. However, homologous antitoxin remains in the serum for over 4 weeks after injection, and it is possible that the duration of circulation is a factor of importance in determining the degree of interference with the toxoid. Available evidence (Levine *et al.* 1966; McComb & Dwyer 1963; Rubbo & Suri 1965) shows, however, that simultaneous active and passive immunization in opposite arms with adsorbed toxoid and homologous antitoxin does allow a satisfactory immune reponse.

When simultaneous active and passive immunization is practised there is the possibility that the patient will be left unprotected for the period of time between the disappearance of the passive antitoxin and the development of his own antitoxin. This 'unprotected gap' should not be considered as a significant drawback to simultaneous immunization, since the alternative of delaying the toxoid injection will undoubtedly give rise to a longer 'unprotected gap'. When passive protection is provided by human antitoxin, which has the advantage of prolonged circulation, the unprotected gap may well be completely avoided (e.g. Levine *et al.* 1966).

A further question that should be considered in relation to simultaneous immunization is the possibility that the toxoid might have an adverse effect on the passive immunity by combining with antitoxin and removing it from the circulation. This point has been examined in animal experiments and in man and it is clear that toxoid causes only a slight reduction in the concentration of passive antitoxin in the blood (Bergentz & Philipson 1958).

# 8

# PREVENTION OF TETANUS 4

### *A summarized scheme for tetanus prophylaxis*

It is difficult, if not impossible, to devise a scheme for tetanus prophylaxis with which all authorities would be in full agreement. Nevertheless, on the basis of the considerations we have discussed, decisions must be taken as to which of the various measures should be adopted for the care of the individual patient. It may therefore be helpful to present to the reader a prophylactic scheme that we have found to be practicable.

Since it is true that active immunization is the most effective prophylactic measure, and is the only way of preventing tetanus following trivial or unnoticed injuries, the emphasis of the scheme is placed on active immunization. It should be the responsibility of medical practitioners and of casualty officers to ensure that immunization is initiated in all wounded patients who have not previously been immunized. The importance of completing the course of injections should be emphasized to the patient, and the significance of tetanus immunization explained to him. The patient should also be issued with a card on which is entered the date of each toxoid injection together with the type of toxoid given.

The treatment required by the injured patient is influenced by his immunization history, but the dividing lines between the various immune categories into which patients might fall must, as previously discussed, be decided to some extent arbitrarily. It is unfortunately true that in most countries, at the present time, the majority of the population have never been immunized.

Surgical cleaning of the wound must be considered of prime importance for prophylaxis in both immune and non-immune patients; in any case, surgical débridement is part of the normal wound care procedure which must be practised irrespective of measures that aim specifically at preventing tetanus.

In areas where *tetanus neonatorum* is common, efforts should be made to improve the standard of hygienic care of the mother and the newborn infant. Until hygienic midwifery can be achieved, we advise the active immunization of pregnant women by means of two intramuscular injections of adsorbed toxoid, given 6 weeks apart, since this will prevent neonatal tetanus. A similar scheme is sometimes advocated for patients undergoing elective surgery in hospitals in which post-operative tetanus sometimes occurs. This can undoubtedly be a valuable measure, but it should not be used as an alternative to improving the surgical hygiene.

The most difficult decision concerning prophylaxis is that of choosing between heterologous antitoxin and antibiotics for patients in whom it is necessary to supplement the débridement and for whom human antitoxin is not available. In the absence of field evidence of the relative effectiveness of the two possibilities the choice must be weighted in favour of that which is least likely to be harmful. At the present time, in developed countries, reactions to antibotics are less frequent than hypersensitivity reactions to horse serum, and the position in the developing countries is probably similar, so that antibiotic prophylaxis, properly used, is generally to be preferred to prophylaxis with horse serum.

There are certain patients in whom we recommend that both antitoxin and an antibiotic should be given, because there is experimental evidence that an antibiotic can reduce the amount of antitoxin necessary to protect (Smith 1967). Patients for whom both are recommended are: (*a*) those with very severe, 'tetanus-prone' wounds (p. 39); (*b*) where human antitoxin is not available for patients who have previously had horse serum, but who are judged to require antitoxin again for their present wound. Such patients are liable to eliminate the antitoxin early and may be left unprotected if chemoprophylaxis is not also employed.

TABLE 8.1. Measures for tetanus prevention in the wounded in addition to careful surgical débridement.

| Condition of wound | Measures recommended according to immune status of patient[a] | | |
|---|---|---|---|
| | *A* | *B* | *C* |
| Clean superficial wounds or abrasions seen within 6 hours of injury | None | Toxoid[b] | Toxoid[b] |
| Badly contaminated or infected wounds; wounds with evident devitalized tissue; deep puncture wounds; wounds more than 6 hours old, i.e. the 'tetanus-prone' wound. | Toxoid[b] | Toxoid[b] | 1 Toxoid[b]<br>2 Antibiotic[c]<br>3 Human antitoxin[d] *or* Heterologous antitoxin[e] |
| Other wounds not falling into above categories | None | Toxoid[b] | 1 Toxoid[b]<br>2 Human antitoxin[d] *or* antibiotic[c] *or* Heterologous antitoxin[e] |

*a* Immune status—refers to patients who have had:

*A* Basic immunization course within previous year; *or* a booster injection within previous three years.

*B* Basic immunization course with adsorbed toxoid between 1 and 10 years previously; *or* a booster injection of toxoid more than 3 years previously; *or* only two of the three doses of toxoid of the basic immunization course, within the previous 5 years.

*C* Basic immunization course more than 10 years previously; *or* only two of the three doses of toxoid of the basic immunization course, more than 5 years previously; *or* only one dose of toxoid; *or* unimmunized.

*b* Toxoid = adsorbed toxoid (such as Tet/Vac/PTAP, B.P.). Every effort should be made to complete the course of immunization—i.e. three spaced injections.

*c* Antibiotic—can be (i) penicillin—phenoxymethyl-penicillin capsules (B.P.) 250 mgm 6-hourly for 5 days; or fortified Procaine Penicillin (B.P.) 2·0 ml intramuscularly daily for 5 days; or a mixture of

| | | |
|---|---|---|
| benzyl penicillin | 300 mgm | one dose intra-muscularly; *or* |
| procaine penicillin | 1600 mgm | |
| benzathine penicillin | 600 mgm | |

cloxacillin, 500 mgm, 6-hourly before meals for 5 days;

(ii) tetracycline 250 mgm 6-hourly for 5 days;

(iii) erythromycin 500 mgm 6 hourly for 5 days;

*d* Human antitoxin = 250 units intramuscularly.

*e* Heterologous antitoxin—pepsin refined, 1500 units (Tet/Ser, B.P.). Horse antitoxin is the one most commonly available. To be given only if the patient is not believed to be hypersensitive, i.e. no history of reactions to horse serum and no reaction, general or local, within half an hour of injecting 0·05 ml of the serum subcutaneously.

*Note 1 Patients hypersensitive to horse serum* (i.e. history of previous reactions, or reaction to the trial dose) should NOT be given horse antitoxin. If no human antitoxin is available, bovine or other species of refined antitoxin may be given—provided the patient does *not* react to a test dose.

*Note 2 Patients who have had horse serum on a previous occasion* should be given a further dose only if there is a strong indication, and chemoprophylaxis should also be used.

*Also Note:* The measures referred to concern tetanus prophylaxis only; other procedures may be necessary as part of the wound care itself. For example, antibiotic will probably be required for most patients with infected wounds.

# 9
# CLINICAL FEATURES

There are a number of striking clinical features in tetanus, most of which may be grouped under the terms rigidity and reflex spasms. They make up the characteristic signs of the disease, play the dominant role in diagnosis and will be described before the symptoms.

## *Signs*

*Rigidity* of muscles is usually the first sign. It shows itself in various ways, some or all of which may be present at the same time. Trismus is said to be present when the muscles of the jaw are stiff and the mouth cannot be fully opened, an observation which gave rise to the name 'lockjaw'. Stiffness of the facial muscles alters the expression considerably, a point which is only fully appreciated as a rule later when the patient has completely recovered. The change in expression is most marked when he smiles: a peculiar sneering appearance results from pursing of the lips and retraction of the angles of the mouth. This is the *risus sardonicus*, perhaps the best-known sign of the disease. Involvement of pharyngeal muscles leads to dysphagia, often a troublesome feature and frequently an early symptom. Neck stiffness fixes the head and rigidity of abdominal muscles and those of the back splints the trunk. Sometimes excessive contraction of the long muscles of the back gives rise to opisthotonos, which can be of alarming degree. More often, however, the trunk is straight or only slightly extended and if, as so frequently happens, the legs and arms are also stiff, the patient adopts a peculiar 'ram-rod' posture which helps in the recognition of the disease. Simultaneous rigidity of muscles and their antagonists is characteristic of the disease; a useful way of testing for this sign is to palpate the long muscles of the back and the abdominals bimanually.

In addition to these features, there are others to be added in the case of newborn infants. Arms and legs are usually held slightly flexed, the former being partly crossed over the abdomen with the hands clenched. Quite often, too, the tip of the thumb may be seen protruding between index and third fingers; excessive flexion of the toes is also common. When the infant attempts to cry, the sound he emits is a somewhat stifled one and his face wrinkles up in an exaggerated *risus sardonicus*. Stiffness of pharyngeal muscles and those of the lips impairs sucking. Together with crying, this is commonly the first sign of *tetanus neonatorum* noticed by the mother.

*Reflex spasms* should be clearly distinguished from muscular rigidity. Both are essential features of the fully developed disease. Quite commonly, in milder cases, rigidity is present without spasms; rarely, in neonatal tetanus, spasms may be seen in the absence of rigidity, but this is usually a late manifestation when early rigidity has given place to flaccidity. When spasms occur they are more alarming than rigidity and much more dangerous. Indeed, patients with muscle stiffness alone seldom die, while those with reflex spasms frequently do, as will be seen in a subsequent chapter.

A reflex spasm consists of a sudden exacerbation of the underlying rigidity. There is simultaneous and excessive contraction of muscles and their antagonists, and the posture of the patient is exaggerated. Opisthotonos, for instance, becomes worse, and slightly flexed arms flex a fraction more in a convulsive manner. Both duration and intensity vary. There may be no more than a momentary stiffening of muscle groups, but usually each spasm lasts several seconds and is abrupt in onset and extremely painful. Such spasms may occur spontaneously or they may be excited by some trivial external stimulus.

Sometimes there is a series of spasms following shortly after one another in rapid succession, and in neonates especially a continuous run of them may be observed. Under such circumstances it is not difficult to appreciate that respiration is embarrassed. Adequate pulmonary ventilation is impossible, hypoxia occurs and cyanosis is often seen; and there are good grounds for the belief that if repeated attacks of this sort are allowed to occur, irreversible cerebral damage follows and death becomes inevitable.

Although less important than spasms, several other clinical features of tetanus deserve attention. Fever is a common finding which may be due to the disease itself, to complications or to treatment. It will be dealt with again in later chapters. Sweating occurs frequently; it is sometimes profuse and it may be troublesome. Sinus tachycardia is quite a frequent finding and is occasionally a marked feature of the disease, with occasional pulse-rates in excess of 180 per minute (Vakil *et al.* 1965*a*).

## *Symptoms*

Some authors such as Spaeth (1940) have described premonitory symptoms such as restlessness, insomnia, irritability and headache, but we have not been impressed by their occurrence and doubt whether they play a significant part in diagnosis. Common initial symptoms are stiffness of muscles which may be generalized or regional; pain in the jaws or in the back or neck; and difficulty or pain on swallowing. Not infrequently the patient complains of abdominal pain, pain in the chest or fever. Other symptoms include sweating, a feeling of oppression in the chest and difficulty in breathing. Sometimes spasms constitute the first complaint in tetanus, but whether they occur at the outset or later, they are an extremely painful and alarming experience which the patient soon learns to try to avoid by lying as quietly as possible and speaking only when he has to.

Few patients complain of symptoms related to the portal of entry of the toxin, but this is not surprising when it is remembered that the wound is most frequently a trivial one. In many cases no wound or injury of any kind can be detected. There was no lesion in 21 per cent of the Durban series of 510 children and adults with tetanus, and a comparabile proportion has been recorded by workers in India (Patel *et al.* 1965*a*; Vakil *et al.* 1965*b*). In some patients, however, tetanus follows a major lesion such as an extensive burn, a compound fracture or septic abortion; in such cases the clinical features of the disease are obviously modified.

## *Diagnosis*

With the possible exception of strychnine poisoning, no other condition presents a clinical picture like fully-developed tetanus. There are few diseases with which it can be confused. In the early stages when only trismus is present, there may be difficulty in excluding local causes since the clenched jaws limit proper examination of the mouth. Generally, however, careful examination will reveal increased muscle tone elsewhere, either at the time or a little later. Sometimes predominant neck rigidity demands the exclusion of meningitis; examination of the cerebrospinal fluid in such cases is diagnostic, no changes being present in tetanus. Dislocated jaw may be superficially confused with tetanus. On occasions we have seen nurses with hysteria which was mistaken for tetanus, and tetanus has been incorrectly diagnosed in patients with schizophrenia or encephalitis.

Although diagnosis generally presents no real problem, clinical observations should be thoroughly performed and accurately recorded. They are rather more important than an exhaustive history. Although an adequate history is essential, few patients with the disease in its severest forms are disposed towards answering all the questions normally asked in history-taking; many of them can profitably be left until the patient has been sedated. Nothing is more important than careful observation of the patient for some time without physical examination or disturbance of any sort—not only for diagnosis but also in the assessment of severity upon which prognosis and choice of treatment depend. There should be no hurry to proceed with the examination until the appearance of the patient and his posture have been adequately observed and, in particular, spontaneous spasms have been looked for over a period of time (10 minutes or more may be necessary) and their duration, frequency and severity noted. Palpation confirms the stiffness of muscles which the history and the patient's appearance and posture suggest. Reflex spasms are very painful, and once they have occurred their return is greatly feared. They are often set off by palpation or by other procedures. Examination should therefore be particularly gentle, disturbing the patient as little as possible. Fever and tachycardia may be present, and after a bout of spasms cyanosis may be detected. Tendon reflexes are often brisk but no particular importance is attached to this sign.

Communicating with patients suffering from tetanus is often difficult. Their jaws are frequently stiff when they are first seen, and those who have experienced spasms already fear moving themselves lest these recur. Sedation adds to the difficulty. Nevertheless, few patients clearly remember their illness afterwards, suggesting some alteration in consciousness. In occasional patients distinct abnormalities of behaviour can be observed in the early days of convalescence.

## *Clinical types*

A number of these have been described. *Local* tetanus is a form found in immunized persons in which involvement of muscles near the site of injury occurs, without spreading elsewhere. Much more often, however, the disease is generalized. The term *modified* tetanus has been applied to cases in which the manifestations are damped down by previous immunization. The distinction between *ascending* and *descending* tetanus has already been made: most cases in clinical practice fall into the latter category. Several other terms have been used. *Cephalic* tetanus is a form of the disease occurring in about 1 per cent of cases (Vakil *et al.* 1965*b*) in which there is paresis or paralysis of cranial nerves, usually unilateral and associated with the generalized disease. The seventh cranial nerve is most frequently affected, and sometimes spasms are seen on the opposite side of the face. Ptosis, iridoplegia and external ophthalmoplegia have also been recorded. When tetanus follows abdominal wounds and the bulbar and respiratory muscles are maximally involved, the name *splanchnic* tetanus has been applied. *Puerperal* and *post-abortal* tetanus refer to cases infected through the female genital tract.

Apart from recognition that tetanus in immunized persons generally follows a modified (and favourable) course, the use of these various terms confers no special advantages in regard to clinical assessment or management. By far the most useful classification is a simple one based on the presence or absence of reflex spasms. Patients with muscular rigidity without spasms are considered to have *mild* tetanus, while those with frequent and severe reflex spasms are labelled *severe*. *Moderate* tetanus is the intermediate category for patients with rigidity but only occasional spasms, particularly when these are mild and of short duration. Placing a patient into one of these three types is generally not difficult, but sometimes some hours or even a day or two must elapse before the type of case one is dealing with becomes apparent. Experience has shown that there is a big difference between patients in whom the disease process progresses rapidly from the first symptom (such as trismus) to the establishment of frequent, severe (and dangerous) reflex spasms and those in whom the progression is much slower. This 'march' of the disease forms an important part of the proper clinical assessment of the patient. For its significance to become apparent, consideration must be given to the natural history of the disease.

### *Natural history*

The *incubation period* has been found to vary considerably in those patients in whom a history of injury can be obtained. In the majority the first symptoms come on within 14 days. Short periods of 4 to 6 days are quite common, particularly in neonates, and in many patients there are longer incubation periods of up to a month. Occasionally the incubation period appears to be as short as 1 or 2 days or as long as 3 months. It must be remembered, however, that it is always difficult to be certain that the only obvious lesion present is the source of the infection, or when there have been several recent injuries, which can be incriminated. Too much reliance should therefore not be placed on this observation when it is used as an aid to prognosis.

The first spasms generally occur some hours or days after the first symptoms. This *period of onset* of reflex spasms is a most important observation in tetanus, as Cole (1940) pointed out. In the most severe cases it may be very short indeed, often only an hour or two, and once again short periods of onset are most commonly found among neonates. The rate of spread of the clinical features in tetanus after the first spasm is also important. Generally when the period of onset is short the disease is severe and the severity often increases rapidly, so that the full gravity of the malady reveals itself in hours or a day or two at the most. On the other hand, when the period of onset is a long one, the subsequent progression is usually slow, but this relationship is by no means invariable. In some patients spasms begin a long time after the first symptoms and then increase rapidly in frequency and severity. The period of onset can be fairly accurately expressed in hours, but the progression or 'march' thereafter is an impression largely dependent on the judgement of the clinician.

Despite a wide range of possibilities as regards the natural history of tetanus, many cases behave in a rather similar way. The initial symptoms, such as trismus, pain in the neck or muscle stiffness elsewhere, come on 7 to 10 days after an injury of some sort in children and adults, or after birth in the case of neonates. Within 48 hours the first reflex spasm occurs, followed by the next an hour or so later, probably after a disturbance of some kind. The march of events is now often rapid so that by the next day spasms come on without apparent stimulus and recur at short intervals. The patient is in obvious distress. Secretions collect in the mouth and pharynx which the patient cannot readily swallow, opening the jaws is difficult if not impossible, and clearly painful; speaking is a labour, and movement of any kind is avoided for fear of initiating spasms. Moreover spasms, rigidity of the thorax and the rather tenacious secretions collected about the upper respiratory tract embarrass respiration and, particularly after a bout of uncontrolled spasms, cyanosis may be observed or the patient may stop breathing. In the worst cases fever is high and in some there is profuse sweating. All these manifestations occur while the patient remains conscious, so that his suffering must be profound.

The peak is often reached some 3 days after the first sign, and the disease maintains its gravity for the next 4 or 5 days before its severity begins to wane. In most cases the first 8 days are the worst. In those who survive this period, clear evidence of improvement is present by the tenth day or the twelfth at the latest. Most deaths in tetanus occur before this, as can be seen from reports of several large series of cases treated conservatively. In Spain, Torres Gost and Figueroa-Egea (1965) showed that 60 per cent of deaths occurred within the first 6 days and 90 per cent by the end of the twelfth day. Eighty per cent of all deaths in the Bombay series of over 2000 cases reported by Vakil *et al.* (1965*b*) took place in the first 4 days, and almost 90 per cent of fatalities in the Delhi series of comparable size recorded by Vaishnava *et al.* (1965) were between the first and the eighth day. These recent reports confirm the findings of Spaeth (1940): his own experience and that of others in the United States, giving a total of 614 patients, showed that more than 90 per cent of deaths occur in the first 10 days.

After 10 days not many spasms occur, even in the most severe cases. By the end of 2 weeks most patients are convalescent, suffering only from the inconvenience of residual muscle stiffness. This is manifest by inability to open the mouth fully or by difficulty in swallowing, turning the head, sitting up in comfort or expressing themselves fully in conversation. Frequently there has been considerable loss of weight and the patient feels weak. Three weeks in some and 4 weeks in most patients sees almost complete recovery, but occasionally stiffness may be prolonged beyond this time.

## *Complications*

Respiratory complications are by far the commonest and are probably the most important. It has already been noted that excessive secretions are frequently found in the upper respiratory tract and are sometimes tenacious in character. Their presence is a threat to the lungs. It is not difficult to visualize how readily secretions may be inhaled after a laryngeal spasm or following a bout of generalized spasms. These usually impair chest movements and pulmonary ventilation, and give rise to a feeling of suffocation, and they are succeeded by much deeper breathing for a time after the muscular spasms have passed off. Patchy areas of *atelectasis* are produced if aspiration of several small plugs of mucus occurs, but if, as is sometimes the case, the aspirated material is larger, atelectasis may be more extensive.

Such aspirated material is frequently infected, whether it comes from the upper respiratory tract, as it usually does, or arises from the vomited contents of the stomach, as occasionally happens. Atelectasis can therefore be expected to be followed by infection. This sequence of events is not, of course, the only one leading to pulmonary infection, the combination of enforced immobility and lowered resistance predisposing to bronchopneumonia. Whatever its pathogenesis, however, *pneumonia* is all too common a complication of tetanus.

It is sometimes difficult to tell the difference between these two complications, since the physical signs of bronchopneumonia and scattered areas of atelectasis may be the same and many patients with tetanus are pyrexial from the disease itself. A change in the character of the secretions should alert the clinician to the onset of penumonia. As will be seen in the section on treatment, one of the advantages of the total paralysis regime is that adequate physiotherapy and removal of aspirated secretions are possible and atelectasis may be reversed. In conservatively treated patients, on the other hand, this is not usually possible, and the persistence of collapsed areas of lung must favour the development of pneumonia. The distinction between the two becomes an academic one in such patients, treatment for pneumonia being indicated as soon as signs suggesting atelectasis or pneumonia are detected.

Three other complications in the respiratory system are of great importance. *Laryngeal spasms* cause airway obstruction, inadequate pulmonary ventilation, hypoxia and cyanosis. Death occurs if the spasm lasts long or is not quickly relieved by therapeutic measures. Laryngeal spasms therefore constitute one of the most feared complications of tetanus, particularly since they may occur for no obvious reason in any patient at any time. Usually they take place early on in the disease, but occasionally there is an unexpected laryngeal spasm quite late, when the severest manifestations appear to be over. This dramatic event may even complicate the otherwise favourable clinical course in a patient who until then was judged to have tetanus of mild degree or at most of only moderate severity. Because of this, confidence in the outcome of the disease should always be tempered with caution. Besides following an episode of laryngeal spasms, *cyanotic attacks* and periods of *apnoea* occur as separate complications in many patients with severe tetanus. Both may follow a prolonged bout of generalized spasms. Sometimes, however, patients stop breathing without preceding spasms and for no apparent reason. The heart goes on beating for a time and then slows, and if the apnoeic attack is not observed in time for resuscitation to be undertaken cardiac arrest soon follows.

*Cardiovascular* complications have been recorded in many series, but generally they are overshadowed by those of the respiratory system. Some degree of tachycardia is quite common. Occasionally it may be severe ($>$180/min) as it was in 14 per cent of the 200 consecutive cases intensively studied by Vakil *et al.* (1965*a*), who observed other disturbances of rate and rhythm and detected histological changes in the myocardium. Most commonly these consisted of cloudy swelling but in some cases the changes were considered to be those of toxic myocarditis. Their animal experiments on isolated rabbit heart suggested a direct action of the toxin, which was contrary to the findings of Bronnimann and Stirnemann (1956), who injected animals with large doses of toxin, producing respiratory failure and flaccid paralysis although the heart was almost entirely unaffected.

Several other workers have reported electro-cardiographic changes and observed necropsy evidence of myocarditis in human tetanus (Alhady *et al.* 1960; Smythe 1963; Patel *et al.* 1965*b*) and we have encountered conspicuous tachycardia and had to deal with cardiac arrest in particular. There is therefore no doubt that the heart may be affected by this disease. What is in doubt, however, is whether these abnormalities are due to direct action of the toxin on the myocardium rather than the result of the hypoxia of respiratory failure.

Variations in the blood pressure are of considerable importance. Vakil and his colleagues found hypotension in 29 per cent of their patients and occasionally encountered hypertension. We have long been impressed by a clinical picture in neonates which carries an almost hopeless prognosis among those treated conservatively. The infant is cold and flaccid and, although there are spasms from time to time, the patient is usually seen to be lying limp and almost lifeless. The pulses are difficult to feel; respiration is slow, irregular and often gasping. This state of affairs sometimes goes on for many hours or even for several days before death occurs. Such a picture was reproduced in animals by Bronnimann and Stirnemann after massive doses of toxin. Hypotension and circulatory collapse have assumed prominence as a clinical entity in tetanus since the introduction of the total paralysis regime (Smythe & Bull 1959; Alhady *et al.* 1960; Clifton 1964). Although action of tetanus toxin on the sympathetic nervous system cannot be excluded (Kerr *et al.* 1968), it seems possible that these circulatory changes are some of the more obvious manifestations of endotoxin shock (from gram negative secondary invaders such as *E. coli*) in patients who would otherwise die of overwhelming tetanus intoxication, life being prolonged by the mechanical maintenance of pulmonary ventilation.

*Fractures* occur quite commonly. Radiological changes consisting of compression of the vertebral body with anterior wedging are present in over half of the patients who survive (Veronesi 1956; Wright 1960; Chaubey 1965; Patel *et al.* 1965*c*). The lesions are confined to the thoracic spine. Sometimes one but more frequently several fractures are found, most often of the fourth, fifth and sixth thoracic vertebrae. Multiple lesions are commonplace and as many as nine have been observed. Occasionally the manubrium sterni has been involved as well.

Neonates who survive appear to be less affected than others. These fractures are most frequently seen in children and young adults, but no age is immune. In an analysis of a group of our own patients Wright (1960) showed that the incidence increased markedly with the severity of the disease when judged on the presence or absence of reflex spasms.

A number of theories, toxic, vascular and mechanical, have been put forward to explain the occurrence of vertebral fractures in tetanus. The most striking fact about them is their localization in the mid-thoracic region, and an important point is that similar lesions have been described after various forms of shock therapy (Epstein 1955). Mechanical factors are therefore most likely to be responsible, although a vascular element cannot be excluded. There are two popular mechanical theories. One of them, offered by Roberg (1937), is that the extensor muscles are weakest in the upper thoracic region, the full force of flexion being concentrated there; repeated compressive blows produce collapse, although any one blow on its own might be insufficient to do so. The other theory, advanced by Dietrich *et al.* (1940), points out that simultaneous contraction of flexors and extensors gives rise to longitudinal compression of the spine as a whole, forcibly increasing the natural spinal curves; hyperextension is produced in the lumbar and cervical regions, while there is marked flexion in the thoracic spine. Davis and Rowland (1965) explain the absence of fractures in the lumbar and cervical regions by the fact that both are supported during hyperextension by the neural arches, no such support being offered during the forcible flexion of the thoracic curve. Whatever the precise mechanism, it is clear that spasms in particular, but probably rigidity as well to a lesser extent, flex the thoracic spine about a fulcrum which is situated in the region of the posterior part of the fifth vertebral body or the neural arch and compress the anterior parts of the fifth and adjacent vertebrae.

Despite their frequency these fractures cannot be regarded as an important complication of tetanus. They apparently cause no pain, do not affect prognosis, lead to no neurological sequelae and generally heal without deformity, although sometimes kyphosis results (Quinlan 1954). It seems certain that better control of rigidity and spasms, such as by the total paralysis regime, will diminish the frequency with which they occur.

# 10

# CAUSES OF DEATH

Investigation of the causes of death in tetanus, as listed by most workers who have studied large series of cases, leads to one clear conclusion: morbid anatomical lesions alone do not explain death in every instance. What soon becomes clear, however, is that the respiratory system is involved in the vast majority of patients. Looking at the findings in four large series should suffice to illustrate this point.

Creech *et al.* (1957) attributed death to pneumonia in 42 per cent of 171 patients who died at the Charity Hospital, New Orleans, between the years 1943 and 1956. Other respiratory causes such as atelectasis, aspiration, pulmonary oedema and asphyxia brought the respiratory causes of death up to 78 per cent. The remainder were made up of septicaemia, convulsions, cardiac arrest and unknown causes.

Garcia-Palmieri and Ramirez (1957) list the probable mode of death in 66 patients in their series of 202. Respiratory causes (respiratory failure, pneumonia, laryngospasm and pulmonary oedema) accounted for the majority (61 per cent); in other cases death was believed to be due to toxaemia or to sustained convulsions. There was no apparent cause of death in 7 patients (11 per cent).

Vakil *et al.* (1965) analysed the findings in 602 cases. Cardio-respiratory failure, laryngeal spasms and pulmonary infections accounted for the great majority of deaths (80 per cent). Death was attributed to hyperpyrexia, to the effects of treatment, or to its neglect in others, but no cause could be ascertained in 7 per cent.

Morbid anatomical lesions found at necropsy in 139 cases were recorded by Patel *et al.* (1965). Infections in the respiratory tract were again the commonest findings (49 per cent), bronchopneumonia being the predominant lesion. Myocarditis and intracranial haemorrhage or thrombosis were observed in a few patients and there were other incidental findings, but in a big group (21 per cent) there were no abnormalities at all.

What emerges from these studies and many like them is that the respiratory system figures prominently in lists of apparent causes of death in tetanus and most often bronchopneumonia is incriminated. In a small but definite minority, however, no cause whatever can be detected. The exact contribution of each of the suspected causes of death is more difficult to assess. We attempted this in Durban by critically analysing the necropsy findings in a series of clinical trials of various conservative forms of treatment (Adams 1958). We took particular note of changes in the respiratory system but found histological evidence of pneumonia in less than a third. Small areas of collapse, pulmonary congestion or oedema were sometimes seen, but usually the changes were not striking. Exhaustion as a cause of death did not seem likely, except in neonates, and respiratory obstruction due to laryngeal spasms was only occasionally the terminal event. Most often we found it difficult to be sure what had caused death.

Later on Wright (1960) undertook a detailed analysis of the mode of death in 250 patients from the same unit. There were 179 neonates and 71 children and adults. The neonates could be divided into two groups according to their survival time. Of 69 infants dying less than 48 hours after admission, death was almost always associated with poorly controlled or uncontrollable spasms. The most striking feature at necropsy was intense congestion of the viscera, notably liver, lung and brain; sometimes the right side of the heart was dilated. Mild pulmonary oedema or atelectasis was present in a third of the cases, but bronchopneumonia was detected in only 9 (13 per cent). Quite a different picture was seen among the 110 infants who died at a later stage. Spasms had usually been adequately controlled and many had lived long enough to pass into a cold, flaccid phase with irregular gasping respiration, bradycardia and peripheral cyanosis. Some pulmonary oedema and atelectasis were found at necropsy but congestion was less marked. Aspirated milk was sometimes present. In this group, however, there was much more evidence of bronchopneumonia (42 cases, i.e. 38 per cent), but its extent varied and in only about half of the patients was its severity considered sufficient to have caused death.

Among the 71 non-neonatal patients, death followed poor control of spasms in 26 (37 per cent), also usually within 48 hours of admission. The necropsy findings were similar to those in neonates. In 5 patients laryngeal spasm was the immediate cause of death, although generalized spasms had been controlled; post mortem examination showed oedema of the glottis and extensive atelectasis. As was the case in neonates, penumonia tended to occur largely in those who survived longer than 48 hours. In the whole group, histological evidence of bronchopneumonia was found in 25 patients (36 per cent), in nearly half of whom it was insignificant in extent. Pneumonia appeared to be the major cause of death in only 4 patients; in 10 others it was regarded as a contributory cause. In many patients death could not be adequately explained on the morbid anatomical evidence, but in some of them the preceding clinical events suggested respiratory failure. The temperature and pulse rate would rise and breathing increase in depth and rate, become irregular and then cease. Such episodes of apnoea sometimes occurred in the absence of previous bouts of severe spasms; in one patient who had never had reflex spasms ('mild' tetanus), fatal respiratory arrest suddenly occurred.

There is no doubt that morbid anatomical findings alone do not explain every death in tetanus. Indeed, a convincing explanation is only found in a minority of patients. Exhaustion after uncontrolled spasms has often been invoked as a cause, but in patients having severe and repeated spasms it is much more likely that death is due to the cumulative effects of episodes of hypoxia which undoubtedly accompany generalized spasms.

Whether such effects adequately explain death in all cases is not known, and this raises the question of the role of medullary intoxication. Of particular importance are the changes in the central nervous system observed by Baker (1942, 1943), who reviewed the literature of this somewhat neglected filed in the study of tetanus, showing that opinions were almost equally divided regarding the existence of lesions. His own observations were made on 12 cases. Up to the fifth day of the illness, changes were limited to the nerve cells, which showed mild swelling and chromatolysis. In patients who survived longer, perivascular glial nodules and demyelinization were sometimes present. Of some importance is the case he described in considerable detail (Baker 1943). On admission to hospital the patient showed cardiac and respiratory irregularities, his breathing 'at times being extremely slow or very rapid, shallow and labored and sometimes being normal'. Despite adequate control of spasms, respiratory signs became more marked and he died 'apparently from medullary paralysis'. On histological examination the most extensive neurological involvement was in the motor nuclei of the fifth and the dorsal nuclei of the tenth cranial nerves. Almost every nerve cell was altered; Baker considered the changes in many of them to be permanent and irreversible. In contrast, only minimal changes were seen in the cord; these he regarded as reversible. The well-documented occurrence of apnoeic attacks in tetanus, unrelated to previous bouts of generalized spasms which could themselves be expected to embarrass respiration, added to Baker's findings, justifies the view that medullary intoxication is one of the causes of death in tetanus.

What has been written in this chapter concerns observations on series of cases in which the patients were treated entirely by conservative means. Since the introduction of total curarization and intermittent positive-pressure respiration (I.P.P.R.) uncontrolled spasms as a cause of death in tetanus has disappeared. Respiratory failure still occurs but is much less important; it may follow technical faults (such as a blocked tracheostomy tube) or pneumonia (which lowers the lung compliance and may make adequate ventilation impossible). In many centres pulmonary infections remain a major problem in patients on I.P.P.R. Moreover, some workers have encountered a shock-like syndrome which is frequently fatal (Clifton 1964; Adams *et al.* 1966) and is possibly the result of gram-negative septicaemia. These aspects of the subject are dealt with more fully in the chapter on I.P.P.R. Nevertheless, a striking reduction in the mortality rate has followed the introduction of this regimen. This seems to be because it eliminates, or can significantly reduce, the importance of three of the major causes of death we recognized in patients treated conservatively—uncontrolled spasms, respiratory failure and pneumonia. The frequency with which a fourth cause (irreversible brain-stem damage) occurs is difficult to ascertain, but the remarkable record of successes with the I.P.P.R. regimen in one centre (Leeds), where there were only 7 deaths in 57 consecutive cases (Ellis 1963), suggests that permanent lesions due to tetanus intoxication of the medullary centres occur infrequently. They cannot therefore be regarded as a major cause of death.

The effect of tetanus toxin on autonomic nervous system function has had little study, but recently an association has been shown between various cardiovascular disturbances in severe tetanus and increased levels of catecholamines in the plasma (Keilty *et al.* 1968) and the urine (Kerr *et al.* 1968). These changes consisted of fluctuations in blood pressure (sometimes with episodes of fairly marked hypertension or profound hypotension), vasoconstriction (often with a line of demarcation between peripheral cold and proximal warm areas in the limbs), tachycardia, cardiac irregularities and profuse sweating. Such features may be encountered in cases of severe tetanus, however treated, and often presage death. It is therefore possible that the autonomic nervous system is directly involved in tetanus, but how often this is a major or even a contributory cause of death is not known.

However, when cardiovascular disturbances due to sympathetic autonomic overactivity occur, rational therapy would be the use of an alpha-adrenergic blocking drug, e.g. phenoxybenzamine, to reduce peripheral vasoconstriction and a beta-adrenergic blocking drug, e.g. propranolol, to protect the heart. If chlorpromazine is being used to control spasms there will already be a substantial alpha-blocking effect. Prys-Roberts *et al.* (1969) considered phenoxybenzamine to be too long-acting, although this drug can be used without difficulty in phaeochromocytoma, and substituted the adrenergic-neurone-blocking drug bethanidine. This substitute has the potential disadvantage that it does not block the nerve to the adrenal medulla and also sensitizes to circulating catecholamines. Whether the use of these drugs is of such practical importance as to influence mortality remains unknown for the present as experience has not yet got beyond the anecdotal stage and definitive studies will be difficult.

# 11

# PROGNOSIS

After reviewing the case-histories of all patients admitted with tetanus to the Charity Hospital in New Orleans over a 50-year period, Creech and his colleagues expressed the opinion that 'tetanus is a self-limiting disease the outcome of which is largely determined before treatment can be instituted' (Creech *et al.* 1957). Prior to the introduction of total paralysis and intermittent positive-pressure respiration, few could justifiably contest the validity of this view, and there is still much to be said in its favour.

Many of the prognostic criteria can be elicited from the history or from observation during the early stages of the disease. Particular attention should be paid to them. Some important factors such as previous immunization and the rate of toxin production in the wound are discussed elsewhere in this book. Race, sex, age, the nature and site of the wound, the incubation period, the period of onset, delay in admission to hospital, pyrexia, intercurrent disease, and the presence or absence of reflex spasms have all been listed as prognostic criteria, and their relative importance is worth examining in some detail. It will be seen that two are of little importance, while others play a major role in determining the outcome and must be taken into account when treatment is planned.

In his well-known paper on prognosis, in which the value of the period of onset was stressed, Cole (1940) also drew attention to the higher incidence of the disease in males and the lower mortality rate in women. His numbers were small, however, and his experience in regard to sex differences in death rates* contrary to what has emerged from an examination of many larger series. In their analysis of over 4000 cases in Bombay, Patel *et al.* (1965*a*) found a slightly

* 'Death rate' is used in this and subsequent chapters in conformity with common clinical usage, instead of 'case fatality rate', which is, however, correct.

higher death rate in women which they attributed to the influence of puerperal tetanus. This had also been observed in North-East India by Sanders (1962), who showed the overall female death rate to be significantly higher than that of males, the difference disappearing when infections of uterine origin were excluded. While it is true to say that tetanus has a higher incidence in males, possibly for occupational reasons, other large series from various countries such as Germany (Hübner & Freudenberg 1954), the United States (Creech *et al.* 1957) and South Africa (Adams 1968) confirm that there is no real sex bias as regards mortality in this disease.

There is also no clear evidence that race *per se* influences the prognosis. A comparison of death rates from different parts of the world would be difficult to interpret since there are too many variables, such as possible differences in the virulence of the organism, previous active or passive immunization and the calibre of the medical services. Nevertheless, mortality rates from countries where social and medical conditions are roughly comparable are usually similar when conservative methods of treatment are used—about 35 per cent for children and adults and some 80 per cent in the case of tetanus neonatorum. It therefore seems unlikely that race plays an important part in determining prognosis.

As regards age, there is no doubt that the highest death rate occurs in the newborn. In contrast the mortality rate is generally at its lowest in older children and in young adults, but it rises again progressively with age.

The death rate is also higher when there is pyrexia, even in the absence of infection; in addition, in tetanus neonatorum the prognosis is bad when the temperature is subnormal. Understandably, the outlook becomes worse with intercurrent disease, pneumonia being the commonest and the most dangerous complication.

The type of injury and the site of the wound do not seem to be of much prognostic importance, with one notable exception. Many authors have stressed the dangers associated with tetanus of uterine origin; Adams and Morton (1955), who collected over 300 cases from the literature, gave the mortality rate as almost 90 per cent. In the Durban series the death rate in this type of case was somewhat lower, possibly following the use of the total paralysis regimen in some patients, but comparison with the death rate in tetanus arising from other sites confirms the increased gravity of the disease when the uterus is the portal of entry (see Table 11.1).

TABLE 11.1. Death rate related to site of wound in 449 children and adults

| Site | Number | Deaths | % |
|---|---|---|---|
| Leg | 239 | 85 | 35·6 |
| Arm | 33 | 10 | 30·3 |
| Head | 40 | 12 | 30·0 |
| Uterus | 27 | 19 | 70·4 |
| No wound | 89 | 29 | 32·6 |
| Trunk | 6 | 1 | — |
| Ear | 10 | 2 | — |
| Operation | 5 | 1 | — |
| Total | 449 | 159 | 35·4 |

Some authors have drawn attention to the frequency of tetanus acquired from ear infections and set aside a special category which they have labelled otogenic tetanus. There seems to be no virtue in making this distinction. Almost 20 per cent of all cases of the disease admitted to one Bombay hospital were otogenic and the mortality rate was below average (Patel *et al.* 1965*b*) but others have held contrary views. There is not much point in pursuing the argument regarding the relatively favourable outcome or the reverse in tetanus arising from the ear—nor for that matter from any other site. When faced with a patient with the disease the clinician would be well advised to remember that it is most dangerous in the newborn and that cases of uterine origin tend to be more severe than average, but he should put these generalizations into proper perspective and pay more attention to three prognostic criteria regarding the importance of which there is no dispute. These are the incubation period, the presence or absence of reflex spasms and the period of onset. Each plays a major role in determining the outcome and all three deserve the closest scrutiny when treatment is being planned.

### *Incubation period*

The incubation period is the time interval in days between the injury and the first symptom; in the newborn it is assumed that infection takes place at birth or soon afterwards. It must be appreciated, however, that the spores of *Cl. tetani* may gain entry to the wound at any time after its occurrence and that we cannot know how soon toxin is liberated after wounding—it could presumably be delayed for several days if necrotic conditions developed slowly. Moreover many patients are vague about the date of injury and ignorant about the subsequent care of the wound, particularly in developing countries, and in such patients reliance cannot be placed on the incubation period as an accurate measurement. Nevertheless, it is quite a good guide to prognosis in many cases. Its value was recognized by Osler (1898), and recent large series confirm its usefulness. The dividing line between those with a bad prognosis and those in whom the outlook is relatively favourable has been variously placed from 7 to 10 days. Which of these days is chosen makes little difference because the trend is the same, as shown in Table 11.2: there is no doubt that a short incubation period generally carries a greater risk of death. It is worth making the point, however, that there is still an appreciable mortality rate among patients with long incubation periods.

TABLE 11.2. Death rate in relation to incubation period

| Author(s) | No. of cases | | Death rate (%) |
|---|---|---|---|
| Children and Adults: | | | |
| Garcia-Palmieri & Ramirez (1957) | 127 | 0–10 days | 43·0 |
| | | More than 10 days | 19·6 |
| Adams (1968) | 297 | 0–8 days | 60·6 |
| | | More than 8 days | 24·7 |
| Patel *et al.* (1965a) | 2497 | 0–7 days | 52·5 |
| | | More than 7 days | 32·2 |
| Sahiar (1944) | 223 | 0–5 days | 59·2 |
| | | More than 5 days | 42·1 |
| Neonates: | | | |
| Tompkins (1958) | 135 | 0–10 days | 95·8 |
| | | More than 10 days | 43·7 |
| | | 0–7 days | 98·7 |
| | | More than 7 days | 76·4 |
| Adams (1968) | 956 | 0–8 days | 60·7 |
| | | More than 8 days | 19·0 |

## *Period of onset*

Most patients can recall exactly when the first symptom occurred and it is usually not difficult to ascertain the time of the first spasm. The interval in hours between them is the period of onset. Cole (1940) drew attention to its importance, and subsequent experience has emphasized what a valuable guide it can be. It is probably the best single index of prognosis among the criteria which can be measured. In two large Indian series the mortality rates declined steadily with each successive 24-hour period from over 60 per cent, when the period of onset was under 24 hours, to less than 11 per cent when it exceeded 96 hours (Patel *et al.* 1965*a*; Vakil *et al.* 1965). Most authors have followed Cole in adopting 48 hours as the critical period of onset, as there is a conspicuous difference in periods shorter and longer than this interval, as demonstrated in Table 11.3.

TABLE 11.3. Death rates in relation to period of onset

| Author(s) | Number of cases | Death rate for period of onset: Under 48 hr | Over 48 hr |
|---|---|---|---|
| Children and Adults: | | | |
| Johnstone (1958) | 88 | 69·0 | 30·0 |
| Patel *et al.* (1965*a*) | 3029 | 63·1 | 22·4 |
| Adams (1968) | 357 | 49·0 | 12·7 |
| Neonates: | | | |
| Adams (1968) | 875 | 60·9 | 20·7 |

It is generally true to say that the more severe the symptoms of a disease the sooner the patient is brought to hospital. Huntington *et al.* (1937) drew attention to this in regard to tetanus, and since then others have commented on the usefulness of the 'admission delay' as a guide to prognosis. As might be expected, there is a close correlation with the period of onset (Sanders 1962) and of the two criteria the period of onset is preferred.

## *Spasms*

No single factor compares with the simple test of noting the presence or absence of spasms. The mortality rate rises conspicuously when spasms occur. Indeed, patients with rigidity but no spasms normally recover no matter how they are treated, whereas a very high proportion of those with spasms die, particularly on conservative treatment. Patel *et al.* (1965*a*) clearly demonstrated this contrast in their analysis of over 4000 case-histories—the death rate was 50 per cent when spasms were present but only 2 per cent when there were none. It is also important to take the frequency and severity of the spasm into account. Our experience has shown that an occasional spasm, especially if it is only slight in degree, does not much worsen the prognosis. Although this introduces the undeniable difficulty of precise definition of what is meant by 'occasional' and 'slight', the division of all patients with spasms into two categories seems worth while. When there are many severe spasms the patient is said to have 'severe' tetanus, but when spasms occur only a few times a day and are not as violent in character the term 'moderate' is used. In the Durban series the death rates were much the same in patients with moderate tetanus and in those who had no spasms ('mild' tetanus), and in both categories they were conspicuously lower than the death rate in patients with severe tetanus as we have defined it. This important distinction is shown in Table 11.4. The striking difference in mortality rates between mild and moderate tetanus on the one hand, and severe cases on the other, underlines the overriding importance of spasms, when frequent and severe, in determining the outcome.

TABLE 11.4. Death rate related to severity in 1472 cases (Adams, 1968)

| | Severity | Number | Deaths (%) |
|---|---|---|---|
| Neonates | Mild | 60 | 3·3 |
| | Moderate | 104 | 5·8 |
| | Severe | 798 | 66·0 |
| | Total | 962 | 55·6 |
| Children and Adults | Mild | 74 | 8·1 |
| | Moderate | 122 | 9·0 |
| | Severe | 314 | 50·6 |
| | Total | 510 | 34·5 |

Two more complicated methods of assessing prognosis are those of Patel and Joag (1959) and Phillips (1967). Patel and Joag introduced a grading system, using a number of factors simultaneously. Patients are divided into five grades of severity depending on how many of the following criteria are present: lockjaw; fever within the first 24 hours; spasms; an incubation period less than 7 days; and a period of onset under 48 hours. Fever is defined as 99°F in the axilla or a rectal temperature of 100°F as the minimum levels. Grade 1 consists of patients with only one of these features (generally lockjaw). Each additional criterion alters the grade by one so that when all five are present the severity is regarded as grade 5. In a large series of cases Patel and Joag demonstrated a steady rise in the death rate from none in grade 1 to 83·5 per cent in grade 5. The system clearly has merit, but since it is dependent on the history for two of the criteria it cannot be applied to all cases.

Phillips (1967) suggested a notational system which gave a severity index and enabled the progress of the disease to be recorded numerically. For determining the severity he attached numerical values to different incubation periods, various sites of infection, the immune status and several complicating factors. The course of the disease likewise could be recorded by adding up scores for the severity of spasms, their frequency, the body temperature and various respiratory factors such as the severity of apnoeic attacks. The weight he gave to one or two criteria can certainly be challenged. For instance, he regarded opisthotonos (which may occur without spasms) as graver than whole-body spasms, and he distinguished between different wound sites in what is probably an unjustified way. Moreover, he omits to take the period of onset into account. Nevertheless, this system should not be condemned on one or two points such as these; it clearly attempts to take the whole clinical picture into account.

We prefer the simpler method of relying mainly on the presence or absence of spasms, but we appreciate that there is advantage in taking other factors into account. Thus a patient with severe spasms, in whom the period of onset is long, is likely to fare rather better than one with similar spasms but a short period of onset; and the length of the incubation period should also be considered when judging the probable outcome in this type of case. Generally speaking, the pattern the disease will follow is determined by the state of the patient on admission to hospital and by what happens to him within the first 48 hours. Thus the vast majority of patients diagnosed as severe on admission run a stormy course, while those considered at first as mild or moderate usually continue as such. There are, however, exceptions to this pattern. An occasional patient with severe spasms will settle down on conservative treatment and have infrequent or quite mild spasms after a day or two, unlike the usual course of events in which spasms increase somewhat for a few days and diminish only after 7 or 8 days. Occasionally, too, patients with mild spasms have an unexpected laryngeal spasm or a bout of spasms, or become inexplicably apnoeic days after admission, and such sudden deterioration accounts for the small number of deaths among patients in whom the prognosis seemed very good. Furthermore, the onset of pulmonary complications, particularly pneumonia, adversely loads the chances of recovery as do repeated hypoxic episodes, whatever the cause.

In summary, it can be said that a reasonably accurate assessment of prognosis, in the first place, depends on clinical observation for the presence or absence of spasms and their frequency and severity, but it is important to be prepared to modify the opinion so formed after consideration of the period of onset, the incubation period and other factors such as the occurrence of apnoeic attacks and pneumonia.

# 12

# TREATMENT I

### *General considerations including the use of antitoxin*

Patients with tetanus can only properly be managed in hospital and preferably in special units set aside for the purpose. Even in apparently mild cases it would be very unwise to attempt domiciliary treatment, since the severity of the disease sometimes increases unexpectedly when initially the prognostic criteria (such as a long incubation period and the absence of spasms) seemed to point to a mild course and a favourable outcome.

Satisfactory sedation and reduction of muscular rigidity can usually be achieved at the outset by an intramuscular injection of 50 mg chlorpromazine. This helps to make the patient comfortable and facilitates moving him to hospital. It is better for a doctor to accompany him in the ambulance because emergency measures are sometimes necessary even at this early stage. Two examples are the intravenous administration of chlorpromazine (100 mg) for laryngeal spasm and the treatment of apnoeic attacks. For the latter we recommend manual ventilation using a resuscitation bag which is self-restoring (e.g. the 'Ambubag').

By the time the patient reaches hospital a good idea will have been gained about the march of the disease. Admission without prior diagnosis in the home or place of work, which is often the case in developing countries where the disease is common, necessitates adequate time being allowed for clinical assessment before a regimen of treatment is decided upon. Observing the patient without disturbing him unduly gives information which is quite as important as the history. Initially, exhaustive questioning should be avoided. It will suffice to ascertain the date of the wound, the day and time of the first symptom whether there have been spasms and if so, when the first one occurred. This information, together with the patient's facial expression, his inability to open his mouth fully, and the presence on physical examination of muscular rigidity in the limbs and in the abdominal and back muscles palpated bimanually, usually establish the diagnosis beyond reasonable doubt.

If no spasm has been seen during this time and none has been provoked by gentle examination, the patient should be quietly observed for another 10 minutes or so to see if they occur. Their significance in relation to prognosis has already been stressed. Generally speaking, spontaneous spasms carry a worse prognosis than do those brought on by disturbing the patient in some way. If spasms were reported to have been frequent before the patient was first seen, or if several are observed to occur spontaneously or are caused by mild disturbance, the disease is likely to run a severe course and immediate sedation is mandatory. Spasms are clearly the most dangerous feature of tetanus and care must therefore be taken to avoid provoking them during examination. Even in less severe cases the use of drugs such as chlorpromazine or phenobarbitone will enable a more thorough physical examination to be carried out with less danger to the patient, and they will minimize any discomfort it causes; moreover, such drugs will make the task of taking a full history very much easier.

Patients need not be kept in semi-darkness. This practice was once in vogue, but visual stimuli do not appear to play a significant part in aggravating the symptoms. It is also not certain that auditory stimuli are important in this regard. On the other hand, tactile stimuli usually increase muscle tone and often provoke spasms. Since both are painful and potentially dangerous, a guiding principle in the management of patients with this disease is to disturb them as little as possible. Frequent medical examinations and some nursing procedures, such as repeatedly washing the patient—generally regarded as desirable manifestations of medical and nursing zeal—are best reduced to a minimum in tetanus. Proper attention, however, must be paid to the pulse, the blood pressure, the removal of secretions which collect about the mouth and nasopharynx, the physical signs in the chest and the keeping of intake and output charts.

*Antitoxin.* After adequate sedation, we recommend that all patients should receive at least 10,000 I.U. of equine antitoxin. Therapeutic trials with homologous antitoxin have not been done, but evidence from animals suggests that the dose should be the same (Smith

1967). Preliminary testing for sensitivity is essential except in the newborn, in whom it is unnecessary. Two points mentioned earlier in this book are worth repeating: there is no advantage in giving antitoxin daily over a number of days—one injection suffices (see p. 54), and, after recovery from tetanus, active immunization is necessary (see p. 63).

*Has antitoxin any therapeutic value*? Despite the fact that antitoxin has been in use for many years there is still no unanimity on this point. The reasons are probably threefold:

1 Antitoxin cannot neutralize the toxin that is already acting on the central nervous system (e.g. Webster & Laurence 1963) and a potentially fatal dose may have been fixed in the central nervous system by the time antitoxin is given to the patient.

2 Death probably arises more often from a variety of indirect causes, such as respiratory complications, than from the direct effects of the toxin (see p. 89); such complications may be minimized by skilful supervision of the patient, but they are really a function of the severity of the disease, and this appears to be related to the amount of toxin already fixed in the central nervous system.

3 There are many mild cases that will recover without it and many cases so severe when first seen that death cannot be prevented by anticonvulsants as used in these studies. The benefit may be confined to a comparatively small group, which cannot at present be distinguished from the mass of cases.

It would therefore seem unreasonable to expect a dramatic fall in the death rate from the use of antitoxin as a therapeutic measure.

There have been many uncontrolled studies of antitoxin and expressions of opinion on this question based on experience that is often very large, and opinions differ (e.g. Patel *et al.* 1963, 1965, 1967; Creech *et al.* 1957; Tompkins 1958). These, however, can hardly be regarded as sufficient. The first published attempt to measure the effect of antitoxin according to accepted principles of therapeutic comparison was that of Brown *et al.* (1960). They allocated patients entering University College Hospital, Ibadan, Nigeria, to two groups, so that they received either no antitoxin or 200,000 I.U. of equine antitoxin; the dose was reduced for children. Plainly, to withhold a therapeutic measure where there are theoretical grounds for belief in its efficacy, even though opinion on its merit varies, poses a serious ethical problem. Its justification in this trial was that from time to time supplies were liable to cease for financial reasons, so that patients were sometimes deprived of it in any case. The well-known dangers of injection of heterologous serum provided another reason for avoiding its use if possible. In order to reduce possible loss of life to a minimum it was decided to analyse the results sequentially (Armitage 1960) and to stop the study when a predetermined level of statistical significance had been reached, rather than to perform a fixed sample trial that might result in a needlessly high level of significance being attained. In any case, the choice of numbers for a fixed sample trial presented great difficulties where ignorance of what might be expected was so great.

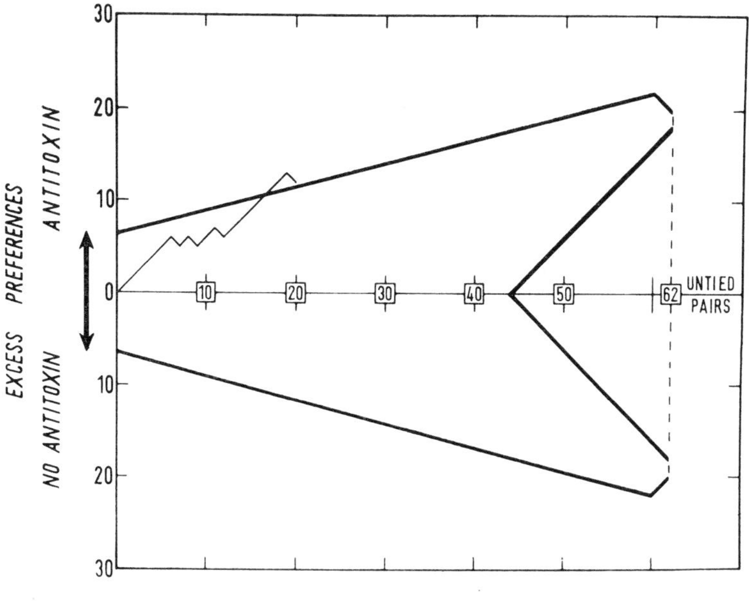


FIGURE 12.1. Sequential chart of a comparison between 200,000 I.U. equine antitoxin and no antitoxin in clinical tetanus. The boundary in favour of antitoxin was crossed at at the 18th preference.

From Brown *et al.* (1960). *Lancet*, 2, 227. (By permission of *The Lancet*.)

In the event the boundary in favour of antitoxin was crossed at the 18th preference (see Figure 12.1), 15 in favour of antitoxin and 3 in favour of no antitoxin. If antitoxin were really ineffective, the probability of crossing a boundary with at least as high a preponderance in favour of one of the treatments, i.e. at an even earlier stage, is less than 0·02. Including the cases that were already entered into the trial at the time the boundary was crossed, and who provided two additional preferences, the trial involved 79 patients.

Following this result, further collaborative studies were organized by one of the authors with colleagues in Ibadan and with others in Bombay. In each trial the dose of antitoxin used in one of the groups was 200,000 I.U., thus preserving a common baseline throughout for comparisons to be made. The results were as follows:

1 200,000 I.U. versus no antitoxin (79 patients): preference for antitoxin (Brown *et al.* 1960).

2 200,000 I.U. versus 500,000 I.U. (270 patients): no preference (Lucas *et al.* 1965).

3 200,000 I.U. versus 50,000 I.U. (293 patients): no preference (Vakil *et al.* 1963).

4 200,000 I.U. versus 20,000 I.U. (300 patients): no preference (Vakil *et al.* 1964).

5 200,000 I.U. versus 10,000 I.U. (796 patients): no preference (Vakil *et al.* 1968).

In the fifth study the discrimination of the design was increased to allow a maximum of 191 preferences instead of the previous 62.

It therefore seems likely that 10,000 I.U. is a sufficient dose. It is preferably given intravenously, for the peak blood level is delayed 48 to 72 hours after intramuscular injection (Turner *et al.* 1958). Because toxin production may be as high in neonates as in adults there seems no strong reason to scale down this relatively low dose for children and neonates, although the latter will, perhaps needlessly, have higher blood and tissue levels.

One other attempt at a controlled comparison of antitoxin versus no antitoxin in patients treated concurrently supports the usefulness of antitoxin (Baker & Grounds 1963) and two more suggest that it has no value (Srivastava & Gulati 1965; Vaishnava *et al.* 1966).

None of the studies mentioned here is beyond criticism and a great deal, relevant and irrelevant, has been written by the various protagonists about different techniques of selection and allocation of patients and analysis of results (see Vakil *et al.* 1968; Patel & Mehta 1967). The details of these discussions are of more interest to the participants than to others and they will not be rehearsed here.

Thus there is no unequivocal certainty as to the value of antitoxin in the treatment of tetanus. It is therefore necessary to consider the results of the statistical studies in the light of knowledge of the pathophysiology of the disease (Laurence & Webster 1963; Wright 1955). When a patient presents with tetanus, some toxin is already fixed to the central nervous system and cannot be neutralized by antitoxin given intramuscularly or intravenously. There is unbound toxin, however, in the blood, in passage up the perineural tissue spaces, in the central nervous system and in the tissues around the site of growth of *Cl. tetani.* This can ultimately affect the central nervous system and so contribute to the severity of the disease. Much of this is accessible to neutralization by antitoxin.

Therefore it is reasonable to suppose that if this accessible toxin is not neutralized the patient may develop the disease more severely than if it is neutralized. Both cost and risk of its use have been invoked as justifying those studies in which equine antitoxin was withheld, but the risk is not, in fact, great, for deaths due to anaphylaxis with therapeutic use are rare. Despite the negative results of two studies (Vaishnava *et al.* 1966; Srivastava & Gulati 1965) it seems reasonable to advocate that antitoxin should be part of the routine treatment of tetanus. All the studies quoted are compatible with the explanation that antitoxin has a slight beneficial effect on the overall mortality, but this effect is not easy to detect.

If antitoxin is to be used it is desirable that the minimum effective dose should be given; the trials described above suggest that 10,000 I.U. equine antitoxin is enough.

The value of local infiltration of antitoxin at the wound site, where this is known, is uncertain, though large amounts of toxin may be present in the tissues at the site of infection (Wright 1955). The clinical value of intrathecal antitoxin is similarly unproved, although there is evidence in its favour from experiments on animals. However, one clinician has stigmatized the arguments for its use as being those of a geographer, based on propinquity, not of a physician, based on physiology (Wainwright 1926). Whatever may ultimately prove to be the case, the meningeal reactions caused by heterologous serum can be serious, and in any further experiments suitable preparations of human antitoxin should be used.

*Feeding.* Patients with mild or moderate tetanus can generally swallow satisfactorily and may be able to take fluids and food orally throughout their illness. The food should preferably be given in semi-liquid form. If there is any difficulty, however, it is better to pass a nasogastric tube and embark on tube-feeding than risk aspiration and consequent pneumonia. The latter danger can also be minimized by close attention to the mouth and nasopharynx, removing the secretions which so commonly collect there through a catheter by means of suction.

Patients with severe tetanus usually require nasogastric feeding from the start. The tube should be passed after sedation. If difficulty is experienced in doing so, intravenous chlorpromazine (100 mg) sometimes helps. If the tube still cannot be passed without provoking laryngeal, oropharyngeal or generalized spasms, it is wise to give up the attempt and rely entirely on intravenous feeding for some days before again trying to pass the tube.

It is important to watch the intake and output of fluid carefully, no matter how patients are fed, since their ability to excrete water is impaired (Holloway 1966). In the case of adults the volume of fluid prescribed for the day should be approximately equal to the amount of urine passed over the previous 24 hours together with 300–600 ml, which will allow for insensible fluid loss. Attention to detail is particularly important in feeding neonates, almost all of whom require a nasogastric tube. Absorption is often poor, so that it is imperative to keep a gastric balance chart. Before each feed the stomach contents are aspirated by syringe attached to the tube, the amount noted and put back together with the difference between this volume and that calculated for the whole feed (see Mann *et al.* 1963). If there is an increasing gastric residue it is wise to reduce the volume of the feed or stop tube-feeding altogether, replacing it for a time by intravenous therapy. During the recovery phase, the Belcroy feeder has proved a useful intermediate between tube-and bottle-feeding, the nasogastric tube being removed as soon as possible because it interferes with swallowing.

*Gastrostomy*, practised by some with enthusiasm, seems to have insufficient advantages over tube-feeding to justify its adoption as a routine.

*Injections.* The frequency of intramuscular injections may give rise to problems in neonates, and sometimes injection abscesses occur, especially if paraldehyde is used. It is therefore important to observe proper precautions and insist on a regular rotation of injection sites.

*Care of the wound.* Decisions about the management of the wound should be based on accepted surgical principles, such as removal of foreign bodies and excision of necrotic tissue. There is no place for radical excision (unless there are strong local indications) since evidence is lacking that this procedure lessens the severity of tetanus once symptoms and signs have appeared. In any event, most wounds are minor ones, so that apart from dressings, surgical interference is the exception rather than the rule.

As regards *post-abortal* tetanus, the same principle applies. Hysterectomy is certainly not justified on the grounds that it will modify the course of the disease. Digital removal of retained products may be done at the time of the first gynaecological examination; anti-gas gangrene serum should be given if retained products or necrotic tissue are present. If dilatation and curettage is necessary, it is probably better to await recovery from tetanus before anything is done, unless there are good gynaecological reasons for interfering at an earlier stage.

In the case of tetanus neonatorum, the *umbilical cord* or the *umbilicus* if the cord has already separated, should be treated conservatively, since there is no justification for the radical procedure of umbilectomy. Quite often the umbilicus is dry when the infant is admitted. If not, a satisfactory practice is too clean the stump with hydrogen peroxide, remove any foreign material and apply mercurothiolate.

*Relief of pain.* Patients with tetanus generally retain full consciousness and therefore suffer considerably from pain associated with the increased muscle tone and the spasms. For its relief it is tempting to give powerful analgesics, such as morphine, but these are best avoided because of the danger of depressing respiration and because they are capable of stimulating the spinal cord. Suffering can be minimized by gentle handling by the medical and nursing staff and by controlling rigidity and spasms. This is attempted in the conservative management of the disease by means of drugs, the sedative action of which generally enables patients to lie quietly or to sleep between spasms. Patients treated by total paralysis and intermittent positive-pressure respiration are, of course, completely relieved of pain. Some sedation, however, is wise, and for this purpose we have used sodium amylobarbitone and chlorpromazine, either of which is a convenient drug to give. After curare has been withdrawn, stiffness often returns; for its alleviation chlorpromazine (up to 50 mg 6-hourly) is most useful.

*The significance of pyrexia.* A number of authors have related the height of the fever to the prognosis (e.g. Vaishnava *et al.* 1965), but several different factors are probably involved, in most cases including marked muscular rigidity and repeated spasms (producing much heat which is often inadequately dissipated by copious sweating), respiratory tract infections and sometimes serum reactions. Nevertheless, there seems little doubt that fever may occur in tetanus in the absence of such causes. We have often observed prolonged pyrexia in patients with severe tetanus who were well controlled by drugs or were on the total paralysis regimen, in whom no complicating infection could be detected and serum reactions were most unlikely. In such cases a variety of antibiotics given empirically has made no difference to the persistence of fever, which usually only begins to abate when the severest phase of the disease is over, and to disappear during convalescence. Under these circumstances fever is less helpful than usual in leading to the detection of complications, although a sudden increase in temperature may give a useful clue.

Respiratory complications are particularly dangerous in tetanus and may be difficult to recognize. In diagnosis there are two particularly important points—changing secretions and changing signs on auscultation.

Abnormal signs in the chest are in any event quite common during the course of the disease. When coarse crepitations with a bubbling quality are heard, they are likely to come from fluid in the upper respiratory tract or from the larger bronchi; when secretions are tenacious in these sites, rhonchi may also be heard, their pitch probably reflecting the size of the tube involved. In such cases change of posture and aspiration generally abolish them. It is very important, however, to look closely at the aspirate and keep a record of its appearance. When the secretions become thicker and change colour to grey, yellow or yellowish-green, the trachea is certainly infected. It is worth while to start culturing the aspirate at regular intervals when this occurs. If signs of pulmonary infection follow, it is a reasonable assumption that the same organisms which have been isolated already are responsible, and the appropriate antibotic can be given until fresh culture results are available.

Fine crepitations, on the other hand, have much more significance than those just described. They mean either collapse or pneumonia. If change of posture in conservatively treated patients, or physiotherapy (percussion and vibration) after suction in patients on the total paralysis regimen do not alter their character or abolish them altogether, the diagnosis is more likely to be pneumonia than collapse, and appropriate treatment should be instituted.

As a physical sign in tetanus patients on I.P.P.R., bronchial breathing is particularly difficult to interpret: the machine and its connecting tubes alter the breath sounds so that we have often been misled. Nevertheless, alteration or disappearance of what sounds like bronchial breathing after physiotherapy and suction also point to collapse as the cause rather than pneumonia.

Another point is worth making about the chest signs of patients on mechanical respirators. The sound of coarse crepitations may emanate from the connecting tubes, and before auscultating they should be checked for the presence of fluid, which can be readily drained by manipulation.

Radiographs generally are not as helpful as might be expected: moving patients with tetanus to the X-ray department is out of the question, and bedside units, which often give films of poorer quality, must be relied upon. In any event, the distinction between collapse and pneumonia is not an easy one to make.

Many authors have recommended the use of penicillin in all cases to prevent infections, a routine which we adopted for a number of years without noting any real benefit. Another argument in favour of the use of penicillin as a routine is that it is capable of killing tetanus organisms. Despite this possible advantage, it is at present our practice to await indications of probable infection and then give penicillin. We also obtain blood cultures when infection seems likely, and we have the aspirated secretions cultured if they thicken or change colour. If pathogenic organisms are found they are, of course, tested for sensitivity to various antibiotics. When there are signs of probably infection in the chest this helps in the choice of antibotic.

The detection and treatment of pulmonary complications is discussed later (see p. 128).

*Fractures* of the vertebral bodies occur when control of spasms has been poor, but they are generally not apparent until the recovery phase of the disease when muscular rigidity is wearing off. If kyphosis is observed at this stage, fractures in the mid-dorsal region are the probable cause and radiological confirmation should be sought. In the newborn, as a rule the spine will straighten out satisfactorily. In older patients, resting on a flat bed during convalescence encourages healing with minimal deformity, but in some cases a spinal brace is advisable when the patient first becomes ambulant.

# 13
# TREATMENT 2

### *Conservative treatment*

This chapter deals with the management of the rigidity and spasms of tetanus using antispasmodic drugs without recourse to tracheostomy or paralysing the muscles of respiration—the so-called conservative treatment of the disease.

There is no doubt that many drugs will achieve some measure of control of both rigidity and spasms, but considerable doubt exists as to whether this results in an appreciable reduction in the death rate. Much of the relevant literature consists of reports of the results of treating small numbers of cases with various anticonvulsant or relaxant drugs; most of them show little regard for the criteria which, as already pointed out, play so important a part in determining the outcome. Even in the majority of the larger studies, where numbers might be expected to minimize the defects inherent in small series, particularly when scant attention has been paid to prognostic criteria, the methods of treatment employed seldom remained constant for long and controls were conspicuous by their absence. Under such circumstances, claims that one regimen is superior to another do not survive careful scrutiny when the effect on the death rate is used as the yardstick for comparison.

In the past, few authors have shown the candour of Creech and his colleagues in New Orleans. Reviewing their experience with 558 cases of tetanus over a 14-year period at the Charity Hospital, they concluded that none of the newer methods could justifiably be claimed to be a therapeutic advance (Creech *et al.* 1957). They showed that there had been a steady decline in the mortality rate for the disease at their hospital over the past 50 years, which they attributed to improvements in the general supportive care of patients rather than to any specific measures. They criticized reports of small numbers of cases such as that of Forbes and Auld (1955), who had 15 successive survivors, for the New Orleans workers from their own experience were able to cite 19 successive recoveries from the disease during a year when, however, the overall mortality rate remained unchanged.

These observations clearly point to the need for properly-designed clinical trials in tetanus before the value of a new anticonvulsant drug can be assessed (Adams 1958). Although several such trials have been undertaken in recent years (e.g. Laurence *et al.* 1958; Adams *et al.* 1959; Hendrickse & Sherman 1966), there is no evidence so far that one drug is better than another as far as its effect on the death rate is concerned. Indeed, the rather cynical view has been expressed that 'any type of sedative or hypnotic agent when properly administered so as to avoid respiratory depression has the same effect or lack of effect upon the outcome of tetanus' (Creech *et al.* 1957).

Nevertheless, conservative treatment cannot be rejected just because there is no clear evidence that it reduces the death rate. There can be no doubt that it affords some measure of symptomatic relief to almost all patients suffering from the disease. While it is true to say that the more radical regimen of total paralysis and intermittent positive-pressure respiration does represent a definite therapeutic advance, as will be shown in the next chapter, it carries undoubted hazards of its own and should only be attempted in specialized respiratory units. Moreover, we do not believe that all patients need such treatment. We have already drawn attention to the small risk of death among patients without reflex spasms ('mild' tetanus), and in our opinion they are best treated conservatively, even when the total paralysis method is available. Tetanus, however, is commonest in the developing countries, most of which are in the tropics or subtropics. Health services in general are inadequate and it is unlikely that specialized respiratory units will be established on a large enough scale to serve the needs of the whole population for many years. (Indeed, it is hoped in any event that priority will be given to prevention when funds and staff permit). Anticonvulsant drugs are therefore likely to remain the mainstay in the treatment of tetanus for a very long time. The advantages and disadvantages of various drugs in common use are therefore worth examining.

## *Choice of drug*

O'Beirne (1836) treated 20 patients who had tetanus with 'tobacco, the gum-elastic tube, and croton oil' and claimed success in 11 of them! We are certainly humbled when we look at these results in comparison with our own, obtained as they were more than a hundred years ago by rather strange means. Nevertheless, if drug therapy is attempted today it should at least be rational.

The qualities required of a drug for use in this disease are that it should abolish spasms altogether or conspicuously reduce their severity and frequency without significantly affecting respiration; act quickly; minimize muscular rigidity; depress consciousness slightly; and possess no troublesome side-effects. Such a drug does not exist. Two groups of substances, however, the barbiturates and the phenothiazines, go a long way towards meeting these criteria (Laurence & Webster 1963) and we place them top of our short list.

*Barbiturates.* A number of these have proved useful in tetanus. Probably those most widely prescribed are thiopentone (valuable by the intravenous route when rapid action is required), amylobarbitone sodium (also short-acting for emergency use and given either intramuscularly or intravenously) and phenobarbitone sodium. We regard the last of these as one of the mainstays of medical treatment. Except in mild cases, it should be administered intramuscularly in a dosage ranging from 30 mg (for neonates) to 200 mg (for adults) at intervals not shorter than 3-hourly in adults or 6-hourly in the newborn.

When used alone to control spasms in severe cases the total daily requirement may be very high; respiratory depression and unconsciousness inevitably follow—two undesirable side-effects, since they aggravate hypoxia and encourage the onset of pulmonary complications. Moreover, phenobarbitone is cumulative so that in neonates, where this effect is most obvious, after initially controlling spasms as little as 30 mg daily may suffice for adequate sedation (Laurence *et al.* 1958). Indeed, we have seen many neonates admitted with severe tetanus, which necessitated heavy sedation, pass into a state of cold flaccidity and lie limp with slow respirations for several days before succumbing, presumably due to a combination of over-sedation and hypoxia; in such cases medullary intoxication probably also plays a part in determining the terminal state just described.

While barbiturates may suffice for the management of mild tetanus, it is very difficult to achieve adequate control of spasms in more severe cases without undue depression of consciousness or adverse effects on respiration, and we therefore do not advocate their use alone.

*Chlorpromazine.* At present chlorpromazine must be regarded as the drug of choice in the conservative management of tetanus.

Early reports suggesting its value came from Cole and Robertson (1955), who combined it with phenobarbitone; from Gelfand (1955); and from Kelly and Laurence (1956), who demonstrated its efficacy experimentally and successfully used it alone in a boy with severe tetanus. Subsequently, randomized clinical trials were designed to compare it with phenobarbitone in neonates and in children and adults using the death rate as the yardstick (Laurence *et al.* 1958). Phenobarbitone was chosen for this comparison because it seemed at the time to have given as good results as any drug (e.g. Forbes & Auld 1955). No statistically significant advantage emerged.

Nevertheless, chlorpromazine is a most useful drug. Given intramuscularly in a dosage of 50 mg 4- or 6-hourly, it relaxes the rigidity and minimizes the frequency of the spasms in many cases without troublesome side-effects. Moreover, when given intravenously (100 mg), it can be valuable for emergency use, and in our opinion replaces the rapid-acting barbiturates. With its aid, a bout of continuous spasms can often be brought under control, and laryngeal or oro-pharyngeal spasms may sometimes be effectively terminated. In milder cases and during recovery from severe tetanus, whether managed conservatively or by the total paralysis regimen, oral chlorpromazine (25 mg to 50 mg several times a day) is recommended for the relief of residual stiffness. This helps the patient to swallow easily and rid himself of secretions about the mouth, and it makes him much more comfortable during convalescence.

Side-effects are minimal provided the total daily dose does not exceed 300 mg. Patients with tetanus are usually kept horizontal or with a mild degree of tilt to keep the head down (facilitating the drainage of secretions from the lungs and their removal from the mouth and naso-pharynx), so the hypotensive effect of chlorpromazine is seldom troublesome. Jaundice is infrequent because the duration of treatment is relatively short. When the muscle bulk is small, as in neonates, some induration due to muscle necrosis may follow, since the drug is irritant in solution, but this has not proved a serious disadvantage if injection sites are taken in strict rotation. It is sometimes tempting to use doses higher than 50 mg in adults, or 12·5 mg in neonates, or to administer the drug more frequently than 4-hourly, because even at these levels spasms cannot be properly controlled. The temptation, however, must be avoided, since larger doses may activate rather than ameliorate the muscle spasms, while reduction of the interval between doses may lead to tachyphylaxis—diminishing response to doses repeated at very short intervals (Laurence & Webster 1961).

*Combination of chlorpromazine and phenobarbitone.* The action of phenobarbitone is potentiated by chlorpromazine, and quite good control of spasms can be achieved without producing toxic effects from either drug by a combination of the two. Cole and Robertson (1955) found it useful to do this when chlorpromazine was first tried in tetanus, and many others since have confirmed the value of using both drugs together. We recommend this form of conservative treatment for all cases of tetanus if curarization and intermittent positive-pressure respiration is out of the question, but we do this because of convenience of administration and apparent lack of toxicity rather than superiority over other regimens in increasing the survival rate. Put to the test in a randomized clinical trial in 96 patients with tetanus, the combination of the two drugs showed no statistically significant advantage over chlorpromazine alone as regards the death rate in the newborn and in older patients (Adams *et al.* 1959).

Adults with severe tetanus should be started on a basic chlorpromazine dosage of 50 mg 4-hourly by intramuscular injection. If control of spasms is still inadequate, occasional injections of phenobarbitone sodium (200 mg) at intervals between those of chlorpromazine will help considerably. We have found that we seldom need to give phenobarbitone more frequently than twice daily. In neonates we reduce the dose of chlorpromazine to 12·5 mg and that of phenobarbitone to 30–60 mg, and we give the former at 6-hourly intervals. For children we use intermediate doses.

We aim to minimize spasms but not to abolish them altogether if the price which has to be paid for this is unconsciousness. We are satisfied if the patient lies quietly, sleeping lightly for much of the time. He may be readily aroused from this state when necessary, e.g. for feeding or injections. At this level of consciousness, respiration and the cough and swallowing reflexes are not unduly depressed, and the risks of hypoxia, atelectasis and aspiration pneumonia are relatively low, although always a danger.

*Diazepam.* This appears to be quite a useful drug in tetanus. Qualitatively similar to its analogue, chlordiazepoxide, it is more potent as a tranquillizer and muscle-relaxant and a much stronger anticonvulsant (Randall *et al.* 1961).

Femi-Pearse (1966) was impressed by its rapidity of action when given intravenously (10 mg) and by its general usefulness when given as a syrup in a dosage of 2–4 mg/kg/day for mild or moderate cases and an average of 9 mg/kg/day for severe tetanus. His report of 6 deaths among 42 cases appears encouraging. In most of his patients, however, he combined diazepam with barbiturates, and frequently used additional procedures such as gastrostomy or tracheostomy—and even intermittent positive-pressure respiration, so that his results are difficult to evaluate.

A randomized clinical trial has helped to establish the place of diazepam in the treatment of tetanus. Hendrikse and Sherman (1966) found that it was relatively ineffectual for the control of spasms (using lower doses than those of Femi-Pearse), although they regarded it as valuable for relieving rigidity. In their series of 149 patients there were no statistically significant differences in the mortality rates of groups of neonates and older children treated by means of a combination of phenobarbitone and chlorpromazine, whether diazepam was added or not (up to 4·4 mg/kg/day).

Diazepam should be regarded as a valuable addition to our short list, since it acts quickly, does not cause respiratory depression, possesses a useful sedative effect, has almost no undesirable side-effects and certainly relieves muscle rigidity.

*Mephenesin.* Since its introduction in 1947, this drug has been used widely (e.g. Veronesi 1956). Mephenesin may be given by mouth, by intramuscular injection, intravenously or per rectum. Its main advantage is that it is capable of stopping spasms, except in the most severe cases, without causing appreciable respiratory depression. When given orally its local anaethetic effect is a nuisance, so it is best administered by stomach tube. It also has disadvantages such as its short action, high dosage, and the fact that it is haemolytic when given intravenously in concentrations above 2 per cent (which reduces its value in an emergency since as much as 500 mg may be needed).

The high doses required—up to 20 g per day—and the difficulties of administration rather than its toxicity or the risk of oversedation limit the usefulness of mephenesin when given alone to control the manifestations of tetanus. It is therefore probably better to use it in combination with other drugs such as chlorpromazine (e.g. Adriani & Kerr 1955) or barbiturates (e.g. Godman & Adriani 1949), but there do not appear to be any good reasons why such combinations should be preferred to that of chlorpromazine and phenobarbitone as described above.

*Meprobamate.* Chemically related to mephenesin, meprobamate has also been used in tetanus, mostly in one centre (Perlstein *et al.* 1960). Like mephenesin, combinations with chlorpromazine and barbiturates have also been recommended. The opinions just expressed about combinations which include mephenesin apply equally here. It may be given by intramuscular injection in doses up to 400 mg for adults, or 100 mg for children at intervals of 3 to 4 hours.

*Paraldehyde.* Previously regarded as the stand-by in tetanus, paraldehyde is no longer extensively used for reasons other than changing fashion. It causes relatively little respiratory depression and can be quite effective for controlling spasms. Average doses are 4 ml to 6 ml for adults by intramuscular injection 4- to 6-hourly. Appropriately smaller doses are given to children down to no more than 1 ml in the case of neonates. Beside the fact that few seem to have claimed its superiority over newer drugs, it cannot be recommended with enthusiasm as the main drug for regular administration in tetanus because it causes induration of muscles and may produce deep sterile abscesses, and difficulty is experienced in finding sufficient injection sites, particularly in neonates. It may be used occasionally, however, or in combination with other drugs such as barbiturates.

*Other drugs. Chloral hydrate* may be given orally to children as background sedation, but has no advantages. The same applies to *bromide*, once used quite frequently but limited by the disadvantage of having to measure blood levels; and to *tribromoethanol*, *methocarbamol* and several other drugs (see Laurence & Webster 1963). *Morphine* and *pethidine* are contra-indicated since they depress respiration and may stimulate the nervous system. Some recent reports indicate that they are still used, but we believe they have no place in the treatment of tetanus.

*Adrenocortical steroids.* Although animal experiments do not suggest that the use of these substances in human tetanus will be effective (e.g. Laurence & Webster 1963), many clinicians have tried them and claimed beneficial results (e.g. Lewis *et al.* 1954). Recently Sanders (1966) reported preliminary studies with betamethasone. The doses he employed were 5 mg to 25 mg per day for children and 10 mg to 55 mg in the case of adults. Although his groups were quite small and the method of allocation to them not stated, he obtained apparently better results when he used betamethasone in addition to sedatives (phenothiazines, phenobarbitone, morphine) than he did in comparable groups of patients who received no steroid but were otherwise managed similarly. Sanders admitted the risks of infection —always a great danger in tetanus—but thought the lower doses of sedatives required for adequate control facilitated proper feeding and were advantageous as regards pulmonary ventilation. Until fuller comparative studies are reported, however, the case for adding steroids to other regimens in the conservative management of patients with tetanus must be regarded as unproven.

*Hyperbaric oxygen.* The place of this interesting but rather elaborate and expensive form of therapy for tetanus cannot be fully assessed on the evidence at present available.

Experiments with mice showed that treatment for an hour in a hyperbaric chamber (at 3 atmospheres absolute) 5 hours after injection of tetanus toxin increased the mean survival time significantly when compared with controls, provided the dose of toxin did not exceed 1·4 m.l.d. (Rö 1965). Rö thought that the toxic effects of oxygen might outweigh any possible therapeutic advantage.

Beneficial results have been claimed in man, but like so many of the reports on the treatment of this disease in which similar claims have been made, the number of patients treated with hyperbaric oxygen in any one series is small, prognostic criteria not sufficiently weighed up, other methods of treatment are used concurrently and controls are lacking (e.g. Pascale *et al.* 1964). A recent paper suggests that the real use of this form of treatment is likely to be for resuscitation after apnoeic attacks rather than as routine therapy (Rhea *et al.* 1967). Rhea and his colleagues treated 10 infants with tetanus neonatorum in a hyperbaric chamber with 100 per cent oxygen at approximately 3 atmospheres pressure for periods usually between 15 and 90 minutes. Four died, an outcome similar to their results with other methods of treatment. Although others have described rapid regression of symptoms and signs when hyperbaric oxygen is used, no obvious effect on the severity or frequency of the spasms was observed in Rhea's series, nor were the requirements for sedative drugs materially affected.

*Neuromuscular blocking agents* may be used to control the spasms of tetanus. Indeed, it appears that Benjamin Brodie suggested the use of *curare* for this purpose in 1811. It was administered to a horse with the disease in 1835 and first used for human tetanus in the 1850s (Poli 1960; Van Bergen & Buckley 1952); surprisingly rational therapy in an era when O'Beirne was using tobacco and croton oil, and in neonatal tetanus the gynaecologist Marion Sims (according to Hartigan 1884) was elevating the occipital bones surgically!

These drugs affect the diaphragm later than other muscles and the intercostals, but in the case of curare it is impracticable to achieve adequate control of the spasms without paralysing respiration (Isacson & Swenson 1941). The use of curare, therefore, only became feasible when artificial means for maintaining respiration were perfected; the total paralysis regimen, which then followed, is discussed in the next chapter.

*Gallamine*, however, has been successfully used without paralysing respiratory movements (e.g. Kamat *et al.* 1958). With this drug there appears to be a greater margin between the paralysis of other muscles and those of respiration than in the case of curare. It has been combined with drugs such as chlorpromazine. Although work with gallamine has not been extensive, it is probable that its safety margin is too low to allow it to be used unless full facilities for controlled respiration are available at the bedside.

# 14
# TREATMENT 3

## *Tracheostomy and intermittent positive-pressure respiration*

It has been shown in previous chapters that the commonest complications in tetanus are respiratory, and that they are responsible for most of the deaths. Uncontrolled spasms may be followed by cyanosis or apnoea; excessive secretions in the trachea or bronchi may impede ventilation, cause atelectasis and encourage the onset of pneumonia; aspirated food has the same effect; and laryngeal spasms or the unexpected development of apnoea may lead to hypoxia and death. In many respects, therefore, tetanus should be regarded as a respiratory problem. The recognition of this fact led to two major developments in the treatment of the disease—tracheostomy alone, and tracheostomy with intermittent positive-pressure respiration (I.P.P.R.).

### *Tracheostomy*

This procedure has much to commend it in many types of respiratory failure. It reduces the dead space by about 100 ml and relieves obstructive laryngeal dyspnoea; it isolates the respiratory tract from the digestive system, and by excluding the chance of aspirating food or gastric juices, reduces the risks of aspiration pneumonia; moreover, it permits the speedy application of controlled ventilation, using mechanical devices should this become necessary.

Tracheostomy was mentioned as a possible means of treating respiratory obstruction in tetanus by Curling in 1837 (Herzon *et al.* 1951). His description was an apt one: 'There is a sense of constriction at the throat, an apprehension of suffocation, and when the paroxysm ensues, all the outward signs of asphyxia are present. I have watched the tetanic patient in the sufferings of this dreadful moment. I have seen him tear away the coverings, grasp his throat with suffused and livid countenance, and in all the agonies of impeded respiration, struggle for breath and for life. In a case of imminent danger from suffocation, it has been suggested that relief might be afforded by an opening made in the trachea.' In our own wards we have occasionally seen such behaviour; some patients, indeed, while fighting to overcome respiratory obstruction have clutched at the throat with such force that the skin has been excoriated and left bleeding.

Tracheostomy would certainly appear to be a logical procedure where secretions are copious or when a laryngeal spasm has occurred and more are feared. It has been advocated for all cases at the beginning of the illness as a means of avoiding such complications and thus lowering the mortality rate. A review of the work of others and an analysis of our own experience, however, shows no conclusive evidence in its favour when it is used in conjunction with a conservative regimen for controlling spasms. Like much of the literature on the treatment of tetanus, opinions on the place of tracheostomy are usually based on small series without adequate controls. In New Orleans, where tetanus is common, Creech and his colleagues admit having been misled in 1950 when they advocated tracheostomy on the strength of a series of six cases, yet their own critical analysis later showed that the drop in tetanus mortality over the 17-year period after its introduction into their clinical practice was similar to that which had occurred in each of the preceding 7-year periods since 1906 (Creech *et al.* 1957).

Before I.P.P.R. became available in Durban in 1959, an attempt was made to assess the place of tracheostomy in the treatment of tetanus neonatorum by conducting a randomized clinical trial on 37 infants, admitting only the most severe cases and using the same standard method of controlling spasms. They were allotted to two groups, in one of which tracheostomy was performed. The trial can be criticized on the grounds that humidification was inadequate, but the conclusion that conspicuous benefit could not be expected from tracheostomy alone seemed justified since the mortality rate was 100 per cent in each group. The death rate among all children and adults with severe tetanus treated conservatively from 1959 to 1965 was found to be virtually the same whether tracheostomy (with humidification) was performed or not (Adams *et al.* 1966). In a separate analysis on the same material, Holloway (1967) showed that infants with tetanus neonatorum but without respiratory failure do uniformly well whether or not tracheostomy is performed, whereas tracheostomy alone (with adequate humidification and proper tracheal toilet) does not alleviate the situation once respiratory failure has occurred, I.P.P.R. being invariably necessary.

*Why are the results of tracheostomy so disappointing*? There is no doubt that this procedure carries special risks of its own: tracheal secretions are increased and the tube may obstruct unless humidification of inspired air is ensured and adequate tube toilet performed; aberrant vessels are sometimes eroded and fatal haemorrhage may follow; the tracheostomy has to be maintained for several weeks until all danger of a laryngeal spasm has passed and during this time, as well as when extubation is attempted, constant vigilance is necessary. Nevertheless, these risks can be minimized by admitting the patient to a unit trained and equipped to deal with these problems. Performing tracheostomy without facilities for proper after-care is clearly unwise. It must be appreciated that tracheostomy *eliminates* only the danger of a fatal spasm of larynx or oropharynx. Unless generalized spasms can be fully controlled the major hazard of inadequate pulmonary ventilation remains. Moreover, apnoeic attacks without preceding spasms may occur at any time and may be fatal.

*When should tracheostomy be performed*? It must be apparent from what has been said that no unequivocal answer can be given. Each patient must be assessed individually. Where no facilities for the total paralysis regimen exist it is wise to adopt a conservative approach. Tracheostomy is not necessary in mild cases, nor should it be performed as a routine when tetanus is severe. In some patients in the latter category, upper respiratory tract secretions are minimal or easily dealt with by suction through the mouth, with appropriate changes in posture; moreover, laryngeal spasms, cyanosis or apnoeic attacks may not occur. Tracheostomy does appear to be indicated, however, for those patients with excessive secretions in the oropharynx that cannot be removed easily because they are too copious or tenacious; and particularly when attempts to do so provoke laryngeal or generalized spasms despite previous sedation. Without tracheostomy, such patients readily develop atelectasis, aspiration pneumonia or respiratory failure, and while there is no proof that it alters the mortality rate, it seems to be a logical procedure.

Some workers have expressed the view that the amount of sedation necessary to control the spasms is reduced after tracheostomy (e.g. Herzon *et al.* 1951). If this is so, the procedure is certainly advantageous, since one of the problems encountered during the management of tetanus by conservative methods is that spasms cannot be controlled in some patients without using a drug dosage which depresses respiration (e.g. when phenobarbitone is employed) or results in other undesirable toxic effects (such as with large doses of chlorpromazine).

Where there are facilities for I.P.P.R. the decision about tracheostomy is less difficult. I.P.P.R. is indicated for all patients who have shown signs of respiratory failure and for patients with severe spasms not properly controlled by sedation. Moderate cases may be tried on conservative treatment without tracheostomy. When a laryngeal spasm has occurred in such patients, however, or secretions are particularly troublesome during the first few days, and in other cases the severity of which is difficult to assess, tracheostomy is a wise step, since it facilitates the immediate application of I.P.P.R. should spasms later become uncontrollable or respiratory failure occur.

### *Intermittent positive-pressure respiration*

During the severe poliomyelitis epidemic of 1952 in Copenhagen, Danish workers developed the technique of tracheostomy with intermittent positive-pressure respiration for patients with paralysis of the muscles of respiration. Later they applied the method to a patient with tetanus, completely abolishing spasms (and respiratory movements) with curare (Bjørnboe *et al.* 1953). Reports of its possible value in children and adults followed from elsewhere, such as Britain (Ablett 1956; Smith 1958) and Nigeria (Glossop & Low 1957), but the death rate in these early series remained high, and controls with which to compare the results were lacking. The earliest report of the use of the method in tetanus neonatorum came from Cape Town, where Smythe and Bull (1959) recorded their experience with 9 neonates, only 2 of whom survived. Nevertheless, since nearly all the evidence regarding the causes of death in tetanus implicates the respiratory system, and since I.P.P.R. offered hope that some or all of the respiratory complications could be avoided, the method appeared full of promise.

Subsequent experience with the newborn has shown beyond

reasonable doubt that these early hopes were justified. A randomized clinical trial on 50 infants with severe tetanus neonatorum, carried out in Durban, showed I.P.P.R. to be superior to a conservative treatment regimen which used phenothiazine derivatives and phenobarbitone to control spasms, the mortality rate being almost halved —from 84 per cent to 44 per cent (Wright *et al.* 1961). A later analysis (Adams *et al.* 1966) appeared to confirm the fact that the method represents a major advance in the treatment of tetanus neonatorum, but it must be pointed out that the comparison is not based on a randomized clinical trial. The death rate in 184 infants admitted consecutively with severe tetanus and managed on the full I.P.P.R. regimen was less than half that of 489 neonates with severe tetanus treated conservatively—36·4 per cent among the former, compared with 78·7 per cent for the latter, the difference again being statistically significant ($P < 0{\cdot}001$). Even better results have been recorded by Smythe (1963) in Cape Town (25 cases, mortality rate 20 per cent) and by Thambiran (1967) in a special series studied in Durban (40 cases, death rate 25 per cent). This striking advance should be viewed against a background of the results of conservative treatment of tetanus neonatorum reported from many parts of the world, in which death rates are almost always in the region of 80 per cent.

In the case of children and adults there is no similar proof. Doubts about the value of the method seemed to be justified by the French report of Mollaret and Pocidalo (1965), who recorded a mortality rate of 64 per cent in their series of 179 patients treated by I.P.P.R. A clinical trial conducted in Durban at the same time, and along lines similar to the neonate trial already referred to, was inconclusive in the case of children and adults. Once the result of the tetanus neonatorum trial was known, the second trial had reluctantly to be stopped after 42 had been treated because some members of the medical and nursing staffs felt it would be unethical to continue. The results, though not statistically significant, were nevertheless encouraging (death rate 43 per cent for the I.P.P.R. group, compared with 67 per cent for the conservative group). In the event, stopping this trial was an unfortunate step. There was no real justification for the assumption that success with I.P.P.R. in neonates, the management of whom in many ways is easier, proved the superiority of the method in older patients. Recent experience in Britain, however, has clearly shown that I.P.P.R. can yield such excellent results in non-neonatal tetanus (59 patients treated consecutively with only two deaths—*Lancet*, 1967) that a comparative trial seeking statistical proof is probably not justified.

*Note on nomenclature.* A number of different names have been given to the method under discussion, such as controlled respiration, controlled ventilation, assisted respiration and intermittent positive-pressure ventilation. It is not our purpose to discuss their relative merits. In this book we use the term 'I.P.P.R.' to denote the regimen of total paralysis with curare and intermittent positive-pressure respiration, and 'assisted respiration' to describe the situation when a paralysing drug is not given at all or is no longer necessary, although intermittent positive-pressure respiration is still applied.

It is our intention to describe these regimens in broad outline, adding some technical details to present a fairly complete picture of the methods employed, the common dangers and the complications. Since it cannot be exhaustive, references will be given to more detailed reports for those who wish to set up respiratory units to treat tetanus in this way. It is appreciated that many centres already have advanced respiratory units with technical expertise beyond that achieved by the workers in the Durban unit, which is geared to manage tetanus on a large scale in an overcrowded general hospital; a situation, we believe, which reflects conditions which are likely to be found wherever tetanus is common.

### *The I.P.P.R. regimen*

After intubation, tracheostomy is performed under local anaesthesia in neonates and general anaesthesia in children and adults. Total paralysis is induced and maintained for 10 days with d-tubocurarine (curare) by intramuscular injection, I.P.P.R. being supplied by a mechanical ventilator. Curare is given in a dosage and at intervals which vary from patient to patient. Generally speaking, it is better to await the appearance of spontaneous movements before giving the next injection than to prescribe curare at regular intervals. Usually the need for another injection of the drug is manifest by the appearance of a few slight jerking movements of the limbs. We have found the average daily requirement of curare to be 212 mg for adults and 14 mg for neonates; suitable doses to start with are 30 mg and 3 mg. respectively.

*Humidification* of the inspired air is essential to avoid crusting of secretions. It can be achieved by blowing the air over water at 100°F (37·8°C) or by nebulizing water into the air stream. Most mechanical ventilators have attachments for this purpose, but we add into the circuit a heat and moisture exhanger, attached between the respirator tubing and the tracheostomy tube (Toremalm 1960). Sometimes the growth of bacteria in the humidification water (particularly *Pseudomonas pyocyanea*) proves troublesome. Continuous pasteurization, achieved by keeping the water at 60°C, will overcome this problem; the inspired air will cool sufficiently if a long connecting tube is used.

*Physiotherapy*. To avoid airways obstruction and to minimize the occurrence of atelectasis and aspiration pneumonia, regular aspiration of secretions is mandatory. It should be done at intervals after physiotherapy to the chest, every hour being desirable. The patient's posture should be altered after each of these sessions. In the case of neonates nursed in a wire-mesh bassinet, nine positions can be achieved—supine, left and right half-lateral with the infant in turn horizontal, head-up and head-down. In the case of older patients fewer positions are possible on an ordinary hospital bed; a tipping bed is therefore an advantage.

It is obviously important to ensure that the patient is not disconnected from the respirator for a period long enough to cause hypoxaemia. A simple way to avoid this danger is for the operator to hold her breath during the whole of the aspiration and to stop the procedure once she experiences discomfort from breathholding. We now use a monitor attached to the chest continuously during I.P.P.R. and adjusted to sound an alarm and show a red light if chest movement ceases for more than 15 seconds.

Because of the danger of hypoxaemia occurring during physiotherapy, it is wise to ensure enrichment of the inspired air with oxygen.

*Auscultation* of the chest is most informative. In particular, the intensity of the breath sounds on the two sides and the appearance of crepitations and their character should be noted. Bronchial breathing is not easy to interpret in patients on ventilators, but attention to the loudness of the sounds and to the type of crepitation yields valuable information about the presence of secretions, their location, and about the onset of collapse or pneumonia. Coarse crepitations point to secretions in the trachea or larger bronchi and are an indication for aspiration, even if it is some time before the regular physiotherapy session is due. Diminished breath sounds on one or other side suggest atelectasis or pneumonia. Atelectasis is the more likely explanation when adventitious sounds disappear or are significantly altered by physiotherapy and aspiration. Persistence of crepitations, on the other hand, suggests the onset of pneumonia.

*Bacterial examination of secretions.* It is wise to observe the aspirated secretions closely for any change in their colour or consistency. Our practice has been to aspirate a specimen from the trachea for bacterial examination at the beginning of I.P.P.R., after tracheostomy has been performed. Thereafter we collect specimens for this purpose whenever there is a change in the breath sounds or when the secretions become thicker. The collection of these specimens must be done carefully, using a sterile catheter and an aseptic technique. It is important that the aspirate is examined and cultured quickly so that the bacterial flora does not change as a result of growth occurring in a warm sputum pot. Observation of temperature changes in tetanus generally does not give a good indication of the onset of pulmonary infection, since pyrexia is common whether infection is present or not.

*An antibiotic*, benzyl/penicillin G, was given to all patients as a routine from the first day of I.P.P.R. early on in our clinical practice, but we now prefer to await some definite evidence pointing to infection. As soon as infection is judged to have supervened, blood is taken for culture and the secretions examined. Bacteriological examination of the blood and aspirated secretions takes time, so antibiotic therapy is started on clinical grounds as soon as these specimens have been obtained. A more appropriate antibiotic judged on sensitivity tests may later be substituted if the infection does not respond to treatment.

*The maintenance of adequate pulmonary ventilation* depends on correct machine settings as well as on the regular removal of secretions and the treatment of atelectasis and pneumonia. Constant vigilance is necessary. The appearance of the patient should be closely watched and the ventilator settings and connections with the tracheostomy tube checked regularly. Continuous medical and nursing attention at the bedside is therefore desirable. Where this is not possible because of a high incidence of tetanus and staff shortages, reliance should be placed on monitoring devices. In some ventilators there are built-in alarm systems to alert the staff against machine failure. Their disadvantage is that they do not detect inadequate delivery of air to the patient. We therefore believe that it is better to be alerted when the chest is not moving properly, which it will not do when the tracheostomy tube becomes blocked, and we accordingly advise the adoption of a chest monitor such as the one described by Eaton *et al.* (1967), the alarm sounding at the bedside as well as in the duty room when the chest fails to move for more than 15 seconds. An added advantage of such a system is that it guards against the danger of disconnecting the ventilator from the patient for more than this period of 15 seconds during aspiration of secretions.

During I.P.P.R. the rate and inflation pressure need adjustment to maintain the $Pco_2$ within normal limits. At the outset the rate may be set between 12 and 15 per minute in adults and at 30 to 37 per minute in the newborn. Initial inflation pressures depend on the machine used, being in the range 10 to 15 cm of water for machines which measure the pressure at zero flow in the mouth (e.g. the Radcliffe respirator) and higher than this (15 mm–20 mm) in the case of ventilators where the measurement is made in the machine (e.g. Bird & Bennett respirators).

Atmospheric air enriched with oxygen is used for all patients. In older patients sweating, tachycardia, a bounding pulse and an elevated blood pressure are useful indicators that there has been a rise in the $Pco_2$; for infants these bedside observations are not so useful. Hypoxaemia is revealed by the detection of cynaosis, but it must be appreciated that this is a crude test. Its appearance calls for immediate action to look for the cause—a blocked tube, excessive secretions, collapse of the lung, pneumonia, leaking connections or faulty machine settings being common—and apply the remedy. What is desirable, of course, is to be able to prevent these gross changes in the blood gases from taking place. Continuous monitoring of the gases is not at present practicable and is probably not necessary.

The first blood-gas estimation need not be done until an hour or so after I.P.P.R. is started, provided ventilation appears to be adequate and the patient's colour remains good. Thereafter one analysis a day will suffice in most cases. A simple method for determining the $P_{CO_2}$, described by Sykes (1960*a*), has been used extensively in our practice. It is a modification of the rebreathing technique of Campbell and Howell (1960); with its aid results can be readily obtained at the bedside using a small rebreathing bag and a simplified Haldane apparatus such as the Aimer model. We managed our patients adequately with good results using this method for some years (Wright *et al.* 1961; Adams 1964); in the newborn a useful addition was the measurement of lung compliance, which is easier to do and acts as a valuable guide to inflation pressures (Jackson 1962; Smythe 1963). Compliance tends to drop somewhat after prolonged I.P.P.R. and higher pressures are required. More recently, the microtechnique for measuring blood-gases described by Astrup has become available. This gives additional information about the blood *p*H and the $P_{O_2}$ and we advise its adoption since it facilitates altering the settings on the respirator as well as the composition of the inspired air. If the $P_{CO_2}$ is found to be high it can usually be corrected by increasing the inflation pressure. If it is normal but the $P_{O_2}$ is low, enrichment of the inspired air with oxygen is necessary. Low $P_{CO_2}$ readings result from hyperventilation, which is easy to correct.

In general it can be said that maintaining $P_{CO_2}$ within the normal range is seldom a problem but the prevention of hypoxaemia frequently is.

*Duration of I.P.P.R.* How long should the period of total paralysis be continued? The period of curarization varies considerably in different centres, and is sometimes continued for several weeks. In the Durban series technical difficulties were encountered when prolonged treatment was attempted. The period of total paralysis was therefore reduced as much as possible and it was found that 10 days was the optimum. Continuing curarization beyond this time would seem, in general, to be unnecessary, since spasms are usually minimal or no longer occur after 10 days, and most deaths in patients treated conservatively take place within this period (see Chapter 9, p. 84). If shorter periods are attempted it is usually found that the disease process is still too active to permit the patient to breathe adequately on his own, and the likelihood of respiratory failure remains. In any event, the respirator has to be kept going to maintain ventilation for a day or two in children and adults and longer in neonates after the last dose of curare, so that the total period of artificial respiration is longer than 10 days. Excessive stiffness of muscles, or the occasional mild spasm after curare has been discontinued, can be controlled by the use of chlorpromazine.

*The tracheostomy and tracheostomy tubes.* It is not within the scope of this book to discuss in detail the technique of tracheostomy nor to compare the various types of tracheostomy tube. The outline given in this section provides a workable plan which is based on experience with many hundreds of patients treated by tracheostomy and I.P.P.R. since 1959.

*Neonates* are allowed to breathe pure oxygen for 10 minutes before 25 mg suxamethonium by intramuscular injection is used to enable the trachea to be intubated with a 3·0 mm Portex tube as a preliminary. The tube is then connected with a respirator, so that tracheostomy can be performed without interference from reflex spasms. After local anaesthesia, two or three tracheal rings are divided through a vertical incision, the oral tube withdrawn a little to facilitate the insertion of the tracheostomy tube and the former kept in place until the latter has been attached to the respirator. A modification of the metal clamp described by Sykes (1960*b*) has been successfully used to secure the tube; a harness is necessary to minimize the danger of the tube being dislodged (see Mann *et al.* 1963 for illustrations and further details).

Following controversy about the relative merits of 'high' and 'low' sites for the procedure, Thambiran (1967) conducted a randomized clinical trial on 40 infants with tetanus neonatorum which showed no significant differences between those with high and those with low tracheostomies as regards the number of deaths, the incidence of complications or the ease of extubation. The practice in the Durban unit has usually been to perform a rather low tracheostomy, between the fourth and sixth tracheal rings.

*Note on tracheostomy tubes in the neonate.* For many years a latex reinforced endotracheal tube, cut to 6·5 cm, was successfully used for I.P.P.R. in Durban (Sykes 1960*b*). The tube was neither curved nor cuffed, a satisfactory fit being achieved by inserting the largest possible size (generally 3·5 mm to 4·0 mm). In an attempt to minimize tracheal damage and therefore facilitate early extubation, a self-inflating tracheostomy tube for neonates was designed and has been extensively tried; it appears to be preferable as regards the incidence of tracheal ulceration and early extubation, and is recommended (Holloway & Thambiran 1967). As soon as the infant breathes on his own, these tubes are replaced by a metal tube, the smallest available being used (such as Parker No. 16). Some workers have successfully used metal tubes throughout.

In *children and adults*, cuffed tubes are desirable. During the period 1959–62 the James tube with a fixed curve was used, but complications (erosion of arteries and anterior tracheal perforations) occurred which justified a search for a better tube for the purpose. A latex armoured endotracheal tube with a cuff and a self-inflating tracheostomy tube have both been successfully used in Durban. As with the newborn, these are replaced by metal tubes as soon as the need for I.P.P.R. has passed. In the case of cuffed tubes it is important to avoid over-inflation of the cuff and to let it deflate at intervals to minimize tracheal damage.

*Weaning the patient from the respirator* starts on the tenth day or the day on which the last dose of curare is given. Vigilance is imperative. Generally speaking, in adults the respirator need not be kept going for more than 24 hours after decurarization commences. The patient's spontaneous respiratory efforts should then be put to the test with the respirator disconnected; spontaneous breathing out of rhythm with the machine and the efficacy of the patient's respiratory efforts during suction give some idea when spontaneous breathing may be tested over a long period. In neonates re-establishment of spontaneous breathing generally takes longer than it does in adults. The period of assisted respiration in the newborn may therefore last 5 days or more. Jackson (1962) introduced a technique for weaning infants from the respirator in which the screw-cap is removed from one arm of the endotracheal connection so that a small aperture opens the tracheostomy tube to the air. Neonates vary considerably in their ability to resume adequate spontaneous respiration from being as good as adults to taking as long as 2 weeks. In each case, therefore, this ability must be put to the test during a period of observation.

*Removal of the tube.* This should not be attempted until at least 2 days after the ventilator has been disconnected.

In *neonates* and *young children* the chances of successful removal at the first attempt are best if the chest is clear and spontaneous respiratory excursions are normal. Pulmonary infections decrease the chances considerably. After removing the tracheostomy tube, the stoma should be sucked clear of secretions and then blocked by putting the finger over the hole to see if the patient can breathe satisfactorily on his own.

In the most favourable cases this becomes quite obvious within a few breaths. The infant in whom the first attempt at detubation will prove successful will go on breathing without any signs of distress; some infants, asleep when the procedure was started, will even continue to sleep, apparently undisturbed.

Others, in contrast, will fight for breath immediately the tube is removed. It must be replaced forthwith. Such patients are most frequently those with respiratory complications, but there is no certainty in prediction.

There are all gradations between these two extremes and the exercise becomes one of trial and error. Our own experience may be helpful in this regard. Some infants, who do well initially, show signs of respiratory embarrassment some hours later, and rib recession is a useful pointer. There is a crucial time, usually the first hour or so after detubation, when the tube can be replaced fairly easily. After this, the track begins to close. If the tracheostomy tube can be replaced through the stoma without undue trauma, this should be done; otherwise intubation via the mouth is necessary. If this nasotracheal tube cannot be removed during the next 2 weeks, tracheostomy will have to be performed for the second time.

In particularly difficult cases we have adopted a technique of attempting to remove the tube at not less than weekly intervals at first, then we try to do so every fortnight, and if still unsuccessful, we increase the interval between attempts to a month or even longer. Patience is rewarded, as a rule, by successful detubation in time—occasionally, it must be admitted, after 6 months or more.

In *older children* and *adults* the situation is quite different: the tracheostomy tube can usually be removed quite easily at the first attempt, even in cases in which there is evidence of chest infection.

### *Other hazards and complications of I.P.P.R.*

It has already been shown that it is difficult to assign a definite cause of death in tetanus, and in the case of the I.P.P.R. regimen this may be even more difficult because of hazards inherent in the method. Most of the factors responsible for death among conservatively treated patients are respiratory, and I.P.P.R. was introduced for this reason. By this means it seemed theoretically possible to minimize the risk of death—perhaps to eliminate it altogether, if the view that tetanus causes irreversible damage to the medullary centres were incorrect. In practice, however, there are a number of hazards and complications. Some of them are due to the fallibility of men and machines, some to infection and some to anatomical considerations. Most of them can be avoided by careful attention to technique.

*Technical faults* can be eliminated by vigilance and by proper maintenance of respirators. The provision of spare machines is essential so that expert workshop inspections can be carried out and repairs done when necessary. In a large unit it is also wise to insist on standard equipment, particularly respirators, since this facilitates maintenance and reduces the chances of mistakes occurring while the staff become acquainted with the attachments and dials of new machines. We, unfortunately, have experienced deaths immediately after the introduction of completely new types of respirator which were attributable to technical unfamiliarity.

Deaths from mechanical faults and from errors of technique are more likely to occur in busy units, where pressure of admissions puts an undue strain on the available medical and nursing staffs. Both need proper training in this type of work. Nurses in particular must know the dangers associated with the method and be aware of the patient's complete dependence for his life on the respirator and the attending staff. This was well put by Smith (1958) when he wrote: 'The fact that the patient is completely paralysed complicates his treatment. He cannot move, breathe or eat and—probably most difficult of all—he cannot communicate.' Doctors, in addition to their usual skills, must be completely familiar with the apparatus and with the significance of changes in the blood-gases. They must be able to replace a dislodged tracheostomy tube and intubate patients with facility. At least one member of the medical staff must be present in the ward day and night and, since a duty roster is inevitable, each doctor must know about the current problems associated with all the patients being treated by I.P.P.R. in the unit.

Two other points are worth making. In a general hospital it is important to ensure that there is a steady turnover of probationer nurses through the respiratory unit rather than a major move of nursing staff at infrequent intervals. One nurse to each patient is desirable but, where this is not possible, the ration should not fall below one to every two patients (excluding the sister and charge nurses). To attempt the I.P.P.R. regimen with insufficient staff is to court disaster.

In concluding this section it seems worth while to add a list of faults that may occur, based on our experience: machine failure; overheating of the humidifier and overfilling of the container when this is of the nebulizer type; detachment of the several connections between respirator and the tracheostomy tube; dislodgement of the tracheostomy tube; and its blockage by copious or encrusted secretions or by blood clot. A wise precaution is to insist on daily routine checking of the apparatus and its connections during I.P.P.R.

*Infection* of the respiratory tract, and in particular pneumonia, is common and a constant worry. Its detection and management have been referred to in previous sections. Control of cross-infection is of major importance; discussion of control procedures is beyond the scope of this book, but reference can be made to other sources (e.g. Williams *et al.* 1966). We attach particular importance to scrupulous aseptic techniques, careful attention to hand-washing, the careful disinfection of respirators and, if possible, the use of disposable plastic gloves when handling tracheostomies. Cross-infection in busy units situated in areas where tetanus is common can be a serious hazard. If it is at all serious it is probably best to stop admitting new patients to the affected ward and to open another ward not recently used for this purpose.

A major hazard in several centres where tetanus is treated by I.P.P.R. has been the occurrence of hypotensive episodes or a state of shock of which hypotension is probably only one manifestation. Hypotension may, of course, follow cardiac arrest or prolonged hypoxia after machine faults or obstructed airways. Apart from these, the patient's condition may be observed to deteriorate some days after the commencement of I.P.P.R. Cold extremities may be noted (often with a fairly definite line of demarcation between distal cold and proximal warm skin), or there may be sweating, tachycardia, hypothermia—especially in the newborn—and hypotension. Like Clifton (1964) and others, we have observed this syndrome in a number of patients, usually with a fatal outcome (Adams *et al.*

1966). These episodes are unlikely to be due to I.P.P.R. itself, because they do not appear to be a problem in other patients (without tetanus) being treated for long periods by this means. Drug reactions can probably be excluded by the variable time intervals observed. We cannot altogether rule out toxic myocarditis, brainstem intoxication or continued activity of the autonomic nervous system (curare abolishes spasms and rigidity but not afferent impulses and autonomic reflexes), but the absence of the syndrome in series of cases from a number of centres, and early on among patients treated in Durban before complicating infections became a major problem, suggest bacteraemic shock as a probable cause.

Since the commoner bacterial causes of pulmonary infections—haemolytic streptococci, pneumococci and staphylococci—can usually be controlled with penicillin or cloxacillin, the cause of intractible infections is not uncommonly found to be multiple-resistant bacteria such as Pseudonomonas, Proteus or other coliform organisms, which may also give rise to bacteraemic shock.

As with bacteraemic shock occurring under other circumstances, poor results usually follow attempts to treat shock associated with I.P.P.R. in tetanus by the use of vasopressors such as noradrenaline. Central venous pressure measurements have not revealed low values in a number of patients who were investigated. It is therefore not surprising that fluid-replacement therapy is not usually permanently effective in reversing the state of shock, unless the causative organism has been isolated and effectively treated with the appropriate antibiotic. Central venous monitoring is advisable if vasodilator treatment with drugs such as phenoxybenzamine or isoprenaline is preferred, fluid-replacement being necessary if the pressure drops below normal. By far the best treatment, however, is to combat infection vigorously, and to anticipate these dangers by careful auscultation of the chest for the appearance of crepitations not affected by aspiration of secretions—which generally means the onset of pneumonia—and by close observation for changes in the quality of whatever is aspirated from trachea or bronchi after physiotherapy. Prevention is most important: attention to aseptic techniques cannot be over-emphasized.

*Distension of the abdomen* occurs not infrequently in neonates. It must be watched for, since the appearance of this sign often heralds danger. Motility of the gastro-intestinal tract is diminished during curarization and gastric emptying time may be delayed. Occasionally paralytic ileus follows. Quite a common cause of distension is constipation, and sometimes there is impaction of faeces, requiring digital removal. These causes can be avoided by nursing techniques which include measuring the gastric residue before each feed, returning this with a volume of milk to make up the balance of the feed (Mann *et al.* 1963) and by the regular use of liquid paraffin. Another cause of abdominal distension is peritonitis, and pneumoperitoneum has been reported (Jackson 1962). Like *pneumothorax*, *pneumoperitoneum* is a rare complication of over-distension of alveoli in babies during I.P.P.R. It is particularly liable to follow manual inflation of the lungs during emergencies (as a means of ventilating with pure oxygen, especially when lung compliance has dropped considerably) or when $P_{CO_2}$ estimations are done by the rebreathing method, or during weighing, if care is not taken with the pressure exerted on the reservoir bag. During over-distension of alveoli, gas passes into the pulmonary vascular sheaths and mediastinal emphysema follows. From here, air may track up into the neck, or it may cause either tension pneumothorax or pneumoperitoneum, or both, requiring emergency treatment by means of the insertion of a needle into thorax or peritoneal cavity, and later using a catheter with under-water drainage (Mann *et al.* 1963).

*Tracheal ulceration* is a very common complication of I.P.P.R. and appears to be particularly important in neonates, in whom direct tracheal inspections may readily be carried out through an auriscope.

Great care must be taken during tracheal suction. Not only must its duration be limited to 15 seconds to avoid severe anoxia and the risk of death, but it must be realized that rough manipulations with the suction catheter may cause ulceration, and bleeding might follow repeated attempts to remove excessive or tenacious secretions.

When latex reinforced tubes are used for neonates, ulceration of the posterior wall of the trachea is almost invariably present in some degree (Thambiran 1967). Sometimes ulceration leads to perforation in older patients as well as in the newborn; occasionally this has led to tracheo-eosophageal fistula or to fatal arterial erosion. In addition to posterior erosions, the proximal anterior tracheal wall is usually depressed by the pressure of the tube. This fact, together with the pooling of secretions trapped above the tracheostomy tube, occasionally results in tracheal stenosis, which is one of the causes of delayed extubation. In addition to posterior ulceration, the tracheal mucosa may be heaped up beyond the end of the tracheostomy tube, and this occurrence as well as the development of granulation tissue in the lumen may lead to tracheal obstruction. Although a curved, self-inflating tube has reduced these risks, they have not been eliminated (Holloway & Thambiran 1967); they are also not uncommon when metal tracheostomy tubes are used (Smythe 1963).

### *I.P.P.R., conservative treatment, tracheostomy: summary of when they should be used*

The mortality rate of patients with severe tetanus (judged on the presence of frequent and severe spasms) is high, no matter what form of conservative treatment is used. In such patients, conspicuous improvement in the chances of survival has followed the use of I.P.P.R., leaving no doubt that it represents a major therapeutic advance.

In contrast, mild or moderate tetanus (no spasms or only an occasional spasm) can be successfully treated in a large majority of cases by conservative means. In view of the dangers of I.P.P.R. on the one hand, and the very good chances of survival on conservative treatment on the other, the latter must remain the method of choice for such patients in most centres.

Performed as a routine on every case of tetanus, tracheostomy (without I.P.P.R.) has not been clearly demonstrated to be advantageous. The procedure, however, is recommended for selected patients in whom the criteria for I.P.P.R. are not present when first seen. Even in the absence of frequent and severe spasms (i.e. 'severe' tetanus), or of respiratory failure, some patients whose tetanus is otherwise judged to be mild or moderate on admission, develop an unexpected spasm of larynx or oro-pharynx, or have secretions about the mouth or upper respiratory tract which are copious or tenacious, or both, and embarrass respiration. Tracheostomy is indicated for such patients. It eliminates the danger of further (and fatal) spasms which obstruct respiration; facilitates the removal of secretions; and permits the immediate application of I.P.P.R. at any time if the spasms become uncontrollable or if respiratory failure occurs.

### *The patient on I.P.P.R.*

There are few reports of what the patient feels during I.P.P.R., but since he is the most important part of the whole procedure (although so far in this account his views have been neglected) it is perhaps appropriate to conclude by quoting extensively from a 'dual account' of an attack of tetanus (Cole *et al.* 1968).*

It was written by a patient and his doctors 'because modern treatment involves uncomfortable manipulations repeated over a period of weeks while the patient is conscious or semiconscious, helpless and paralysed, and unable to explain or protest. During the more difficult phases, particularly soon after tracheostomy and curarisation, or later when reversion to normal breathing is cautiously permitted, the patient is often fully aware of what is going on. For his peace of mind, mutual trust between himself and his attendants should be established as early as possible, by explanation of what is being done. Sedation is helpful but is no substitute for this reassurance.'

The patient, a young analytical chemist, 'would have been classified as a mild case of tetanus but for the disproportionately severe involvement of the muscles of the throat and larynx. This made tracheostomy and artificial ventilation essential at an early stage; for without these measures the risk of choking and aspiration pneumonia was great.

As recorded by the patient, the first symptoms 'consisted in a sudden tightening around my throat causing extreme difficulty in breathing and making swallowing virtually impossible. During this spasm, coughing or expectoration added to the difficulty in obtaining air as my throat seemed to collapse when I tried to inspire.' He could recall his early symptoms well but later his symptoms were only 'snatches of memory'.

Regarding movement he experienced 'a certain amount of discomfort owing to lying in one position. This was definitely helped by being turned over every two hours. Knowing this was to be done brought great relief, and, of course, it was something to look forward to, too. Great discomfort was felt, especially at night when awaking. As far as I can remember this was due to hallucinations at the point of time when the drug was due to wear off. On the whole, comfort could not have been better. A point I am quite sure about is the

* We are indebted to Dr. L. B. Cole for permission to do so.

position of legs. I gained greater comfort when the positions of my legs were varied—e.g., first two hours both straight, second two hours lower one straight, third two hours both bent with thighs horizontal'.

Of major concern were his eyes 'which definitely functioned peculiarly while I was under the drug (tubarine). Firstly, they crossed themselves, giving double vision. Secondly, large objects seemed to be much closer, e.g., when I was lying on my back the ceiling seemed some 18 inches from my nose. The moral here is not to be on one's back. Eyes were improved when I was washed: in fact damp eyes felt normal for a time.'

'Hearing . . . was acute: every sound seemed magnified; I could hear, quite distinctly, the doctors having a good old talk. This was helpful as it occupied my mind—the worst times were when there was nothing to hear. Silence was oppressive, although I realized one couldn't have a continuous noise vibrating through the ward. I'm grateful for the many passages read to me when waking after a nightmare. The radio was also helpful.'

The patient's comments about being taken off the respirator for suction are also well worth repeating. 'After several days I lost the fear of never being able to breathe when off the respirator, as it was always restored quickly. I only had one really scaring time, when the tube fell out after replacement. I know it felt more secure when the tube from the ventilator was *screwed* into the tracheostomy socket and not just pushed in. Also when the tube was taken off before the suction apparatus was made ready, the time taken was terrifyingly long.'

Those who work in respiratory units, so often preoccupied with technical details and routine procedures, would do well to note these points. It is all too easy to assume that the patient paralysed with curare is unconscious because he is immobile—and therefore to ignore him as regards communication. Whenever possible, procedures should be explained to him; and above all, loose bedside talk should be avoided and discussion of prognosis or complications reserved for another place and another time.

# REFERENCES

## CHAPTER 1


BOYD J. (1959). Tetanus in two world wars. *Proc. roy. Soc. Med.*, **52,** 109.

CREECH O., GLOVER A., OCHSNER A. (1957). Tetanus, evaluation of treatment at Charity Hospital, New Orleans, Louisiana. *Ann. Surg.*, **146,** 369.

CULLEN W.H. (1827). *The works of William Cullen*, vol. II, p. 407. Blackwood, Edinburgh.

HILL A.B. (1961). Principles of Medical Statistics. *Lancet*, London.

LOWBURY E.J.L., LILLY H.A. (1958) Contamination of operating theatre air with *Cl. tetani. Brit. med. J.*, **2,** 1334.

POLAND A. (1857). Report of seventy-two cases of tetanus. *Guy's Hosp. Rep.* 3rd series, **3,** 1.

WELLS T. SPENCER (1859). Three cases of tetanus in which 'Woorara' was used. *Proc. roy. med. chirurg. Soc. Lond.*, **3,** 142.


## CHAPTER 2


BATTY I., WALKER P.D. (1964). The identification of *Clostridium novyi* (*Clostridium oedematiens*) and *Clostridium tetani* by the use of fluorescent labelled antibodies. *J. Path. Bact.*, **88,** 327.

BYTCHENKO B. (1966). Geographical distribution of tetanus in the world, 1951–60. A review of the problem. *Bull. Wld Hlth Org.*, **34,** 71.

FEIGEN G.A., PETERSON N.S., HOFMANN W.W., GENTHER G.H., VAN HEYNINGEN W.E. (1963). The effect of impure tetanus toxin on the frequency of miniature end-plate potentials. *J. gen. Microbiol.*, **33,** 489.

FILDES P. (1929). Tetanus VIII. The positive limit of oxidation-reduction potential required for the germination of spores of *B. tetani in vitro. Brit. J. exp. Path.*, **10,** 151.

FRANCIS E. (1914). Laboratory studies on tetanus. *Hyg. Lab. Bull.*, p. 4095. U.S. Pub. Hlth Serv. Govt Printing Office, Washington, 1914.

LOWBURY E.J.L., LILLY H.A. (1958). Contamination of operating theatre air with *Cl. tetani. Brit. med. J.*, **2,** 1334.

MACKIE T.J. (1928). *An inquiry into post-operative tetanus: a report to the Scottish Board of Health.* H.M.S.O., Edinburgh.

MUELLER J.H., MILLER P.A. (1954). Variable factors influencing the production of tetanus toxin. *J. Bact.*, **67,** 271.

NISHIDA S. (1967). Biological properties and toxigenicity of *Clostridium tetani*. Principles on Tetanus. *Proceedings of an International Conference on Tetanus, Bern*, 1966 (Ed. L. Eckmann); p. 111. Huber, Bern.

PILLEMER L., WITTLER R.G., GROSSBERG D. (1946). The isolation and crystallization of tetanal toxoid. *Science*, **103,** 615.

RUBBO S.D., GARDNER J.F. (1965). A review of sterilization and disinfection. Lloyd-Luke, London.

TENBROECK C., BAUER J.H. (1924). Tetanus carriers in experimental animals. *Proc. Soc. exp. Biol. (N.Y.)*, **21**, 267.

WETZLER T.F., MARSHALL J.D., CARDELLA M.A. (1956). Rapid isolation of Clostridiums by selective inhibition of aerobic flora. 1. Use of sorbic acid and polymyxin-B sulfate in a liquid medium. *Amer. J. clin. Path.*, **26**, 418.

## CHAPTER 3

*Brit. med. J.* (1956), *2*, 1478. Stiff man syndrome.

AMBACHE N., MORGAN R.S., WRIGHT G.P. (1948). Action of tetanus toxin on acetylcholine and cholinesterase content of the rabbit's iris. *Brit. J. exper. Path.*, **29**, 408.

AMBACHE N., MELLANBY J. (1965). The mydriatic action of tetanus toxin. Personal communication.

BARNES J.M., TRUETA J. (1941). Absorption of bacteria, toxins and snake venoms from the tissues. *Lancet*, **1**, 623.

BAYLIS J.H., MACKINTOSH J., MORGAN R.S., WRIGHT G.P. (1952). The effect of transection on the ascent of tetanus toxin in the rabbit spinal cord. *J. Path. Bact.*, **64**, 33.

BONNEY J., BOX C., MACLENNAN J. (1938). Tetanus bacillus recovered from the scar ten years after an attack of post-operative tetanus. *Brit. med. J.*, **2**, 10.

BROOKS V.B., CURTIS D.R., ECCLES J.C. (1957). The action of tetanus toxin on the inhibition of motor neurones. *J. Physiol. (Lond.)*, **135**, 655.

D'ANTONA D. (1951). Le tétanos: synthèse théorique et pratique de nos principales connaissances. *Rev. Immunol. (Paris)*, **15**, 93.

FEDINEC A.A. (1967). Absorption and distribution of tetanus toxin in experimental animals. Principles on Tetanus. *Proceedings of an International Conference on Tetanus, Bern*, 1966 (Ed. L. Eckmann); p. 169. Huber, Bern.

FEIGEN G.A., PETERSON N.S., HOFMANN W.W., GENTHER G.H., VAN HEYNINGEN W.E. (1963). The effect of impure tetanus toxin on the frequency of miniature end-plate potentials. *J. gen. Microbiol.*, **33**, 489.

FILDES P. (1929). Tetanus IX. The oxidation-reduction potential of the subcutaneous tissue fluid of the guinea-pig; its effect on infection. *Brit. J. exp. Path.*, **10**, 197.

FIROR W.M., LANWORT A., SHUMACKER H.B. (1940). Studies on the cause of death in tetanus. *Ann. Surg.*, **III**, 246.

FRIEDMANN U., ZUGER B., HOLLANDER A. (1939). The influence of section of the nerve on intramuscularly injected tetanal toxin by circulating antitoxin. *J. Immunol.*, **36**, 485.

GELFAN S., TARLOV I.M. (1959). Interneurones and rigidity of spinal origin. *J. Physiol.* (*Lond.*), **146,** 594.

HOFFMAN F.A. (1879). Ein fall von tetanus traumaticus mit curare behandelt. *Berl. Klin. Woch.*, **16,** 367.

HURST A. (1944). *Medical Diseases of War*, 4th Ed., p. 430. Arnold, London.

HUTTER O.F. (1951). Effect of denervation on local tetanus. *J. Physiol.* (*Lond.*), **112,** 1P.

JANOFF A. (1964). Absorption of tetanus toxin by subcellular fractions of rabbit brain homogenate. *Nature*, **202,** 913.

KELLY R.E., LAURENCE D.R. (1956). Effect of chlorpromazine on convulsions of experimental and clinical tetanus. *Lancet*, **1,** 118.

KRYZHANOVSKY G.N. (1965). On the action of tetanus toxin as a neurotropic agent. *Recent Advances in the Pharmacology of Toxins*, p. 105. Pergamon Press, London.

KRYZHANOVSKY G.N. (1966). *Tetanus*. Medical Publishing House, Moscow.

LAURENCE D.R. (1957). Some observations of drugs in human tetanus. *Clin. Sci.*, **16,** 443.

LAURENCE D.R., WEBSTER R.A. (1958*a*). A method of assaying the antitetanus potency of drugs on experimental local tetanus in the rabbit. *Brit. J. Pharmacol.*, **13,** 330.

LAURENCE D.R., WEBSTER R.A. (1958*b*). The activity of a variety of chemical compounds against experimental tetanus. *Ibid.*, **13,** 334.

LAURENCE D.R., WEBSTER R.A. (1961*a*). Activity of the triethyl analogue of choline in suppressing experimental tetanus. *Lancet*, **1,** 481.

LAURENCE D.R., WEBSTER R.A. (1961*b*). Tachyphylaxis to the antitetanus activity of some phenothiazines. *Brit. J. Pharmacol.*, **16,** 296.

LAURENCE D.R., WEBSTER R.A. (1963). Pathologic physiology, pharmacology and therapeutics of tetanus. *Clin. Pharmacol. Therap.*, **4,** 36.

MELLANBY J., VAN HEYNINGEN W.E. (1967). Biochemical research on the mode of action of tetanus toxoid. Principles on Tetanus. *Proceedings of an International Conference on Tetanus, Bern*, 1966 (Ed. L. Eckmann); p. 177. Huber, Bern.

MEYER H., RANSON F. (1903). Untersuchungen uber den tetanus. *Arch. exper. Path. Pharmak.*, **49,** 369.

PERDRUP A. (1946). Electromyographic investigations on the mode of action of tetanus Aoscia. *Acta pharmacol.* (*Kbh.*), **2,** 121.

PRESS E. (1948). Desirability of the routine use of tetanus toxoid. *New Engl. J. Med.*, **239,** 50.

RANSON S.W., DIXON H.H. (1928). The elasticity and ductility of muscles in the myostatic contracture caused by tetanus. *Amer. J. Physiol.*, **86,** 312.

SCHELLENBERG D.B., MATZKE H.A. (1958). The development of tetanus in parabiotic rats. *J. Immunol.*, **80,** 367.

SHERRINGTON C.S. (1909). *Integrative action of the nervous system*, p. 109. Constable, London.

SOLANDT D.V., PARTRIDGE R.C., HUNTER J. (1943). Effect of skeletal fixation on skeletal muscle. *J. Neurophysiol.*, **6,** 17.

STEER J.C., HORNEY F.D. (1968). Evidence for passage of cerebrospinal fluid along spinal nerves. *Canad. med. Ass. J.*, **98**, 71.

TEALE F.H., EMBLETON D. (1920). The paths and spread of bacterial exotoxins with special reference to tetanus toxin. *J. Path. Bact.*, **23**, 50.

WEBSTER R.A. (1962). Site of action of chlorpromazine and mephenesin in experimental tetanus. *Brit. J. Pharmacol.*, **18**, 150.

WEBSTER R.A. (1965). Effects of mephenesin and chlorpromazine on motor nerve discharges in the rabbit. *Ibid.*, **25**, 270.

WEBSTER R.A. (1967). The effects of tetanus toxin on motor nerve activity in the rabbit. *Int. J. Neuropharmacol.*, **6**, 207.

WRIGHT E.A., MORGAN R.S., WRIGHT G.P. (1950). Tetanus intoxication of the brain stem in rabbits. *J. Path. Bact.*, **62**, 569.

WRIGHT E.A., MORGAN R.S., WRIGHT G.P. (1951). The movements of toxin in the nervous system in experimental tetanus in rabbits. *Brit. J. exper. Path.*, **32**, 169.

WRIGHT E.A., MORGAN R.S., WRIGHT G.P. (1952). The site of action of toxin in local tetanus. *Lancet*, **2**, 316.

WRIGHT G.P. (1953). Nerve trunks as pathways of infection. *Proc. roy. Soc. Med.*, **46**, 319.

WRIGHT G.P. (1955). Neurotoxins of Clostridium Botulinum and Clostridium Tetani. *Pharmacol. Rev.*, **7**, 413.

## CHAPTER 4

BYTCHENKO B. (1967). Tetanus as a world problem. Principles on Tetanus. *Proceedings of an International Conference on Tetanus, Bern,* 1966 (Ed. L. Eckmann); p. 21. Huber, Bern.

EBISAWA I. (1967). Mortality of tetanus in Japan. *Ibid.*, p. 71.

HEREDIA A.F. (1965). Prevention of tetanus in cold surgery in the tropics. *Proc. Int. Conf. Tetanus,* 1963 (Ed. J.C. Patel); p. 640. Bombay.

LOWBURY E.J.L., LILLY H.A. (1958). Contamination of operating theatre air with *Cl. tetani. Brit. med. J.*, **2**, 1334.

MACKAY-SCOLLAY E.M. (1959). An outbreak of post-operative tetanus. *Proc. roy. Soc. Med.*, **52**, 110.

MARTIN-BROUYER G. (1967). Umbilical tetanus. Principles on Tetanus. *Proceedings of an International Conference on Tetanus, Bern,* 1966 (Ed. L. Eckmann); p. 555. Huber, Bern.

PATEL J.C., KALE P.A., MEHTA B.C. (1965). Otogenic tetanus: study of 922 cases. *Proc. Int. Conf. Tetanus,* 1963 (Ed. J.C. Patel); p. 158. Bombay.

REY M., ARMENGAUD M., MAR I.D. (1967). Tetanus in Dakar. Principles on Tetanus. *Proceedings of an International Conference on Tetanus, Bern,* 1966 (Ed. L. Eckmann); p. 49. Huber, Bern.

SERGEEVA T.I., MATVEER K.I. (1967). Geographical distribution of *Clostridium tetani* in the soil of the U.S.S.R. *Ibid.*, p. 77.

SURI J.C. (1967). The problem of tetanus in India. *Ibid.*, p. 61.

VAKIL B.J., AIYER S.N., TULPULE A.T., MEHTA A.J., TULPULE T.H. (1965). A study of 2130 cases of tetanus with special reference to incidence, clinical types and prognosis. *Proc. Int. Conf. Tetanus*, 1963 (Ed. J.C. Patel); p. 54. Bombay.

VERONESI R. (1967). Epidemiology of tetanus. Principles on Tetanus. *Proceedings of an International Conference on Tetanus, Bern*, 1966 (Ed. L. Eckmann); p. 43. Huber, Bern.

## CHAPTER 5

ANWAR A.A., TURNER T.B. (1956). Antibiotics in experimental tetanus: *in vitro* and *in vivo* studies. *Bull. Johns Hopk. Hosp.*, **98,** 85.

BRUCE D. (1920). Tetanus. Analysis of 1458 cases which occurred in home military hospitals during the years 1914–1918. *J. Hyg.* (*Lond.*), **19,** 1.

COX C.A., KNOWELDEN J., SHARRARD W.J.W. (1963). Tetanus prophylaxis. *Brit. med. J.*, **2,** 1360.

EDSALL G. (1959). Specific prophylaxis of tetanus. *J. Amer. med. Ass.*, **171,** 417.

FILLER R.M., ELLERBECK W. (1960). Tetanus prophylaxis. *Ibid.*, **174,** 1.

GARROD L.P. (1958). The chemoprophylaxis of gas gangrene. *J. roy. Army med. Cps.*, **104,** 209.

LINDBERG R.B., NEWTON A. (1954). Sensitivity to antibiotics of *Clostridia* from Korean battle casualties. *Antibiotics Annual 1954* (Ed. Welch H. and Marti-Ibanez F.); p. 1059. Medical Encyclopaedia Inc., 1955.

LOWBURY E.J.L. (1967). *Symposium on Tetanus in Great Britain*, Leeds (Ed. M. Ellis); p. 100.

LUCAS A.O., WILLIS A.J.P. (1965). Prevention of Tetanus. *Brit. med. J.*, **2,** 1333.

IDSØE O., GUTHE T., WILLCOX R.R., DE WECK A.L. (1968). Nature and extent of penicillin side-reactions, with particular reference to fatalities from anaphylactic shock. *Bull. Wld Hlth Org.*, **38,** 159.

MCDONALD R.T., CHAIKOFF L., TRUANT J.P. (1960). An analysis of prophylactic measures in experimental tetanus. *Surg. Gynae. Obstet.*, **110,** 702.

MACKIE T.J. (1928). *An inquiry into post-operative tetanus: a report to the Scottish Board of Health.* H.M.S.O., Edinburgh.

NOVAK M., GOLDIN M., TAYLOR W.I. (1949). Tetanus prophylaxis with penicillin-procaine. *Proc. Soc. exp. Biol.* (*N.Y.*), **70,** 573.

PATEL J.C., POWAR V.F., MEHTA B.C. (1965). Prophylaxis of tetanus in out-patients department. A study of 4000 cases. *Proc. Int. Conf. Tetanus* (Ed. J.C. Patel); p. 649. Bombay.

RUSSELL D.S. (1927). Tetanus V. The local fate of tetanus spores inoculated into guinea-pigs. *Brit. J. exp. Path.*, **8,** 377.

SCHEIBEL I., ASSANDRI J. (1961). Experimental investigation into *in vitro* sensitivity to antibiotics of some field strains of *Cl. tetani. Acta path. microbiol. scand.* Supp., 144, **51,** 249.

SCHEIBEL I., LENNERT-PETERSEN O. (1958). Effect of antibiotics on germinating spores of *Cl. tetani in vitro* and *in vivo*. *Acta path. microbiol. scand.*, **44**, 222.

SMITH J.W.G. (1964). Penicillin in prevention of tetanus. *Brit. med. J.*, **2**, 1293.

TINKLER A.E., SHANNON R. (1966). Daily penicillin serum concentrations following injection of 2·4 mega-units of 'all-purpose' penicillin. *Bull. Wld Hlth Org.*, **35**, 357.

TURNER G.A. (1895). The successful preventive treatment of the scourge of St Kilda (tetanus neonatorum) with some considerations regarding the management of the cord in the new-born infant. *Glasg. med. J.*, **43**, 161.

## CHAPTER 6

BARDENWERPER H.W. (1962). Serum neuritis from tetanus antitoxin. *J. Amer. med. Ass.*, **179**, 763.

BARR M., SACHS A. (1955). Army pathology advisory committee report on the investigation into the prevention of tetanus in the British Army. *W.O. Code No. 1162*, War Office, London.

BAZY M. (1914). Note statistique sur le tétanos. *C.R. Acad. Sci.* (*Paris*), **159**, 794.

BERGENTZ S.F., PHILIPSON L. (1958). Studies on combined tetanus prophylaxis in humans. *Acta. chir. scand.*, **116**, 58.

BIANCHI R. (1962). On serum prophylaxis of tetanus. *Helv. med. Acta.*, **29**, 38.

BINNS P.M. (1961). An analysis of tetanus prophylaxis in 3455 cases. *Brit. J. prev. soc. Med.*, **15**, 180.

BRUCE D. (1920). Tetanus. Analysis of 1458 cases which occurred in home military hospitals during the years 1914–18. *J. Hyg.* (*Lond.*), **19**, 1.

BUFF B.H. (1960). Fatal anaphylactic shock; following intradermal skin test with dilute horse serum tetanus antitoxin. *J. Amer. med. Ass.*, **174**, 1200.

COOKE J.V., JONES F.G. (1943). The duration of passive tetanus immunity and its effect on active immunization with tetanus toxoid. *Ibid.*, **121**, 1201.

COX C.A., KNOWELDEN J., SHARRARD W.J.W. (1963). Tetanus prophylaxis. *Brit. med. J.*, **2**, 1360.

DIXON F.J., BUKANTZ S.C., DAMMIN G.J. (1951). The effect of sensitization and X-radiation on the metabolism of $I^{131}$ labelled proteins. *Science*, **113**, 274.

EDSALL G. (1959). Specific prophylaxis of tetanus. *J. Amer. med Ass.*, **171**, 417.

FILDES P. (1929). Tetanus, ch. X. A system of bacteriology in relation to medicine. Vol III. *M.R.C.*, H.M.S.O., London.

FRANCIS G.E., HAWKINS J.D., WORMALL A. (1957). The use of radioactive isotopes in immunological investigations. 10. The fate of some intravenously injected native proteins in normal and immune rabbits. *Biochem. J.*, **65**, 560.

FULTHORPE A.J. (1957). Tetanus toxin titration by haemagglutination. *J. Hyg.* (*Lond.*), **55**, 382.

GLENNY A.T., HOPKINS B.E. (1922). Duration of passive immunity. Part I. *Ibid.*, **21**, 142.

GODFREY M.P., PARSONS V., RAWSTRON J.R. (1960). Rapid destruction of antitetanus serum in a patient previously sensitized to horse serum. *Lancet*, **2**, 1229.

*Lancet* (1966), **2**, 489. The prevention of tetanus. Statement approved by the International Conference on Tetanus, Bern, 1966.

LAURENT L.J.M., PARISH H.J. (1952). Serum reactions and serum sensitivity tests. *Brit. med. J.*, **1**, 1294.

McCOMB J.A. (1964). The prophylactic dose of homologous tetanus antitoxin. *New Eng. J. Med.*, **270**, 175.

McCOMB J.A., DWYER R.C. (1963). Passive-active immunization with tetanus immune globulin (human). *Ibid.*, **268**, 857.

MACLENNAN R., SCHOFIELD F.D., PITTMAN M., HARDEGREE M.C., BARILE M.F. (1965). Antitoxin response of pregnant women to adjuvant and plain toxoids. *Bull. Wld Hlth Org.*, **32**, 683.

MADSEN E. (1936). The course of the passive immunity after treatment with anti-diphtheria horse serum in rabbits and man. *Acta. path. microbiol. scand.*, **13**, 106.

MOYNIHAN N.H. (1955). Serum sickness and local reactions in tetanus prophylaxis. A study of 400 cases. *Lancet*, **2**, 264.

NOCARD E. (1897). Sur la sérotherapic du tétanos chez les animaux. Essais de traitment préventif. *Bull. Acad. Med.* (*Paris*), **38**, 107.

PARISH H.J., CANNON, D.A. (1961). *Antisera, Toxoids, Vaccines and Tuberculins.* 5th Edition. Livingstone, Edinburgh.

POPE C.G. (1963). Development of knowledge of antitoxins. *Brit. med. Bull.*, **19**, 230.

PORTER R.R. (1963). Chemical structure of $\gamma$-globulin and antibodies. *Ibid.*, **19**, 197.

REGAMEY R.H. (1953). Effets, chez le lapin, d'injections répétées de serum antitétanique issu d'animaux appartenant à des espèces différents. *Schweiz. Z. allg. Path.*, **16**, 873.

REISMAN R.E., ROSE N.R., WITEBSKY E., ARBESMAN C.E. (1961*a*). Serum sickness II. Demonstration and characteristics of antibodies. *J. Allergy*, **32**, 531.

REISMAN R.E., ROSE N.R., ARBESMAN C.E. (1961*b*). Immunologic studies of serum sickness from bovine antitetanus toxin. *J. Amer. med. Ass.*, **176**, 114.

RUBBO S.D., SURI J.C. (1962). Passive immunization against tetanus with human immune globulin. *Brit. med. J.*, **2**, 79.

RUBINSTEIN H.M. (1962). Studies on human tetanus antitoxin. *Amer. J. Hyg.*, **76**, 276.

SMITH J.W.G. (1967). Comparison of the effectiveness of homologous and heterologous tetanus antitoxins. Principles on Tetanus. *Proceedings of an International Conference on Tetanus, Bern,* 1966 (Ed. L. Eckmann); p. 519. Huber, Bern.

SURI J.C., RUBBO S.D. (1961). Immunization against tetanus. *J. Hyg. (Lond.)*, **59**, 29.

TASMAN A., HUYGEN F.J.A. (1962). Immunization against tetanus of patients given injections of antitetanus serum. *Bull. Wld Hlth Org.*, **26**, 397.

TRINCA J.C., REID J.C. (1967). Prevention of tetanus by antitoxin of bovine origin. *Lancet*, **1**, 76.

TURNER T.B., VELASCO-JOVEN E.A., PRUDOVSKY S. (1958). Studies on the prophylaxis and treatment of tetanus. II. Studies pertaining to treatment. *Bull. Johns Hopk. Hosp.*, **102**, 71.

WEIGLE W. O. (1957). Elimination of $I^{131}$ labelled homologous and heterologous serum proteins from blood of various species. *Proc. Soc. exp. Biol. (N.Y.)*, **94**, 306.

## CHAPTER 7

BARR M., SAYERS M.H.P., STAMM W.P. (1959). Intradermal T.A.B.T. vaccine for immunization against enteric. *Lancet*, **1**, 816.

BERGENTZ S.F., PHILIPSON L. (1958). Studies on combined tetanus prophylaxis in humans. *Acta chir. scand.*, **116**, 58.

DAVIES J.R., WRIGHT E.A. (1955). The specific precocious protective action of tetanus toxoid. *Brit. J. exp. Path.*, **36**, 487.

ECKMANN L. (1963). *Tetanus prophylaxis and therapy*; p. 108. Grune & Stratten, New York and London.

EDSALL G. (1959). Specific prophylaxis of tetanus. *J. Amer. med. Ass.*, **171**, 417.

EDSALL G. (1967). Diphtheria, tetanus, and pertussis immunization. *Arch. environm. Hlth*, **15**, 473.

ERICSSON H. (1948). Studies on tetanus prophylaxis. *J. clin. Path.*, **1**, 306.

EVANS D.G. (1943). Persistence of tetanus antitoxin in man following active immunization. *Lancet*, **2**, 316.

EVANS D.G. (1965). Tetanus prophylaxis. *Proc. roy. Soc. Med.*, **58**, 228.

EVANS D.G., SMITH J.W.G. (1963). Response of the young infant to active immunization. *Brit. med. Bull.*, **19**, 225.

FURSTE W., SKUDDER P.A., HAMPTON O.P. (1966). Prophylaxis against tetanus in wound management. *J. Trauma*, **6**, 516.

GOTTLIEB S., MCLAUGHLIN F.X., LEVINE L., LATHAM W.C., EDSALL G. (1964). Long-term immunity to tetanus—a statistical evaluation and its clinical implications. *Amer. J. pub. Hlth*, **54**, 961.

GOTTLIEB S., MARTIN M., MCLAUGHLIN F.X., PANARYO, R.J., LEVINE L., EDSALL G. (1967). Long-term immunity to diphtheria and tetanus: a mathematical model. Principles on Tetanus. *Proceedings of an International Conference on Tetanus, Bern*, 1966 (Ed. L. Eckmann); p. 307. Huber, Bern.

LEVINE L., MCCOMB J.A., DWYER R.C., LATHAM W.C. (1966). Active-passive tetanus immunization. Choice of toxoid, dose of tetanus immuneglobulin and timing of injections. *New Engl. J. Med.*, **274**, 186.

LONG A.P., SARTWELL P.E. (1947). Tetanus in the United States Army in World War II. *Bull. U.S. Army med. Dep.*, **7**, 371.

McCOMB J.A., DWYER R.C. (1963). Passive-active immunization with tetanus immune globulin (human). *New Engl. J. Med.*, **268**, 857.

McCOMB J.A., LEVINE L. (1961). Adult immunization. II. Dosage reduction as a solution to increasing reactions to tetanus toxoid. *Ibid.*, **265**, 1152.

MACLENNAN R., SCHOFIELD F.D., PITTMAN M., HARDEGREE, M.C., BARILE M.F. (1965). Antitoxin response of pregnant women to adjuvant and plain toxoids. *Bull. Wld Hlth Org.*, **32**, 683.

MILLER J.J. Jr., RYAN M.L., BEARD R.R. (1949). Speed of the secondary immune response to tetanus toxoid with a review of war reports and observations on simultaneous injection of toxoid and antitoxin. *Pediatrics*, **3**, 64.

MINISTRY OF HEALTH (1963). *Active immunization against infectious disease.* H.M.S.O.

NEWELL K.W., LEHMANN A.D., LEBLANC D.R., OSORIO N.G. (1966). The use of toxoid for the prevention of tetanus neonatorum. Final report of a double-blind controlled field trial. *Bull. Wld Hlth Org.*, **35**, 863.

PEEBLES T.C., LEVINE L., ELDRED M.C., EDSALL G. (1969). Tetanus toxoid emergency boosters: a reappriasal. *New Engl. J. Med.*, **280**, 575.

PEELER R.M., KADULL P.J., CLUFF L.E. (1965). Intensive immunization of man: evaluation of possible adverse consequences. *Ann. intern. Med.*, **63**, 44.

REPORT (1967). Principles on Tetanus. *Proceedings of the International Conference on Tetanus, Bern*, 1966 (Ed. L. Eckmann); p. 576.

REPORT (1968). National Communicable Disease Center. Tetanus Surveillance. U.S. Dept Hlth, Educ., Welfare.

RUBBO S.D. (1966). New approaches to tetanus prophylaxis. *Lancet*, **2**, 449.

RUBBO S.D., SURI J.C. (1965). Combined active-passive immunization against tetanus with human immune globulin. *Med. J. Aust.*, **2**, 109.

SCHEIBEL I., BENTZON M.W., CHRISTENSEN P.E., BIERING A. (1966). Duration of immunity to diphtheria and tetanus after active immunization. *Acta path. microbiol. scand.*, **67**, 380.

SMITH, J.W.G. (1964). Simultaneous active and passive immunization of guinea-pigs against tetanus. *J. Hyg.* (*Lond.*), **62**, 379.

SNYDER H.E., EDSALL G., LEVINE L. (1966). Tetanus immunization. *J. Trauma*, **6**, 529.

TRINCA J.C. (1963). Active tetanus immunization: effect of a reduced reinforcing dose of adsorbed toxoid on the partly immunized reactive patient. *Med. J. Aust.*, **2**, 389.

TRINCA J.C. (1965). Active immunization against tetanus: the need for a single all-purpose toxoid. *Ibid.*, **2**, 116.

WHITE W.G., BARNES G.M., GALL D., SMITH J.W.G. (1967). Unpublished results.

WHITE W.G., MORRIS-OWEN R., GALL D., SMITH J.W.G. (1968). Unpublished observations.

WHITE W.G., UNGAR J. (1967). Practical aspects of tetanus prophylaxis in a factory population. Principles on Tetanus. *Proceedings of the International*

*Conference on Tetanus, Bern,* 1966 (Ed. L. Eckmann); p. 401. Huber, Bern.

## CHAPTER 8

SMITH J.W.G. (1967). Symposium on Tetanus in Great Britain (Ed. M. Ellis); p. 77. The United Leeds Hospitals.

## CHAPTER 9

ALHADY S.M.A., BOWLER D.P., REID H.A., SCOTT L.T. (1960). Total paralysis regime in severe tetanus. *Brit. med. J.*, **1**, 540.

BRONNIMANN R., STIRNEMANN H. (1956). Experimental tetanus by tetanus toxin and the effect of curare alkaloids. *Proc. Wld Cong. Anaesth.*, p. 282. Burgess, Minneapolis.

CHAUBEY B.S. (1965). Veterbral compression in tetanus. *Proc. Int. Conf. Tetanus,* 1963 (Ed. J.C. Patel); p. 226. Bombay.

CLIFTON B. (1964). Hypotension associated with tetanus. *Lancet,* **1**, 785.

COLE L. (1940). The prognosis of tetanus. *Lancet,* **1**, 164.

DAVIS P.R., ROWLAND H.A.K. (1965). Vertebral fractures in West Africans suffering from tetanus. A clinical and osteological study. *J. Bone Jt Surg.*, **47**, 61.

DIETRICH H.F., KARSHNER R.G., STEWART S.F. (1940). Tetanus and lesions of the spine in childhood. *Ibid.*, **22**, 43.

EPSTEIN B.S. (1955). *The spine. A radiological text and atlas,* p. 333. Henry Kimpton, London.

KERR J.H., CORBETT J.L., PRYS-ROBERTS C., CRAMPTON SMITH A., SPALDING J.M.K. (1968). Involvement of the sympathetic nervous system in tetanus. *Lancet,* **2**, 236.

PATEL J.C., MEHTA B.C., GOODLUCK P.L. (1965*a*). Tetanus: experience with 4718 cases. *Proc. Int. Conf. Tetanus,* 1963 (Ed. J.C. Patel); p. 1. Bombay.

PATEL J.C., GOODLUCK P.L., SHESHIA S.S., DESHPANDE D.H. (1965*b*). Morbid anatomical lesions in tetanus. *Ibid.*, p. 303.

PATEL J.C., MEHTA M.M., GOODLUCK P.L. (1965*c*). Vertebral fractures in tetanus. *Ibid.*, p. 239.

QUINLAN A.G. (1954). Post-tetanic kyphosis. *J. Bone Jt Surg.*, **36**, 80.

ROBERG O.T. (1937). Spinal deformity following tetanus and its relation to juvenile kyphosis. *Ibid.*, **19**, 603.

SMYTHE P.M. (1963). Studies on neonatal tetanus and on pulmonary compliance of the totally relaxed infant. *Brit. med. J.*, **1**, 565.

SMYTHE P.M., BULL A. (1959). Treatment of tetanus neonatorum with intermittent positive-pressure respiration. *Ibid.*, **2**, 107.

SPAETH R. (1940). A clinical study of tetanus. *Amer. J. Dis. Child.*, **60**, 130.

TORRES GOST J., FIGUEROA-EGEA (1965). Mortality in tetanus. *Proc. Int. Conf. Tetanus,* 1963 (Ed. J.C. Patel); p. 86. Bombay.

VAISHNAVA H., PASSEY M.N., NEOGY C.N., GUPTA S.C., DIXIT N.S., ARORA N. (1965). Clinical study of tetanus in Delhi for a period of 22 months. *Ibid.*, p. 33.

Vakil B.J., Mokashi J.M., Tulpule T.H., Shah S.J., Gaitonde B.B., Kazi J., Chabrai N.I. (1965*a*). Cardio-circulatory disturbances in tetanus. A clinico-experimental study. *Ibid.*, p. 255.

Vakil B.J., Aiyer S.N. Tulpule A.T., Mehta A.J., Tulpule T.H. (1965*b*). A study of 2130 cases of tetanus with special reference to incidence, clinical types and prognosis. *Ibid.*, p. 54.

Veronesi R. (1956). Clinical observations on 712 cases of tetanus subject to four different methods of treatment. *Amer. J. med. Sci.*, **232,** 629.

Wright R. (1960). *The treatment of tetanus.* M.D. Thesis, University of Cape Town.

## CHAPTER 10

Adams E.B. (1958). Clinical trials in tetanus. *Proc. roy. Soc. Med.*, **51,** 1002.

Adams E.B., Holloway R., Thambiran A.K., Desai S.D. (1966). Usefulness of intermittent positive-pressure respiration in the treatment of tetanus. *Lancet*, **2,** 1176.

Baker A.B. (1942). The central nervous system in tetanus. *J. Neuropath. exp. Neurol.*, **1,** 394.

Baker A.B. (1943). Medullary intoxication in tetanus. *Amer. J. Path.*, **19,** 709.

Clifton B. (1964). Hypotension associated with tetanus. *Lancet*, **1,** 785.

Creech O., Glover A., Ochsner A. (1957). Tetanus: evaluation of treatment at Charity Hospital, New Orleans, Louisana. *Ann. Surg.*, **146,** 369.

Ellis M. (1963). Human antitetanus serum in the treatment of tetanus. *Brit. med. J.*, **1,** 1123.

Garcia-Palmieri M.R., Ramirez R. (1957). Generalized tetanus: analysis of 202 cases. *Ann. intern. Med.*, **47,** 721.

Keilty S.R., Gray R.C., Dundee J.W., McCullough H. (1968). Catecholamine levels in severe tetanus. *Lancet*, **2,** 195.

Kerr J.H., Corbett J.L., Prys-Roberts C., Crampton Smith A., Spalding J.M.K. (1968). Involvement of the sympathetic nervous system in tetanus. *Ibid.*, **2,** 236.

Patel J.C., Goodluck P.L., Sheshia S.S., Deshpande D.H. (1965). Morbid anatomical lesions in tetanus. *Proc. Int. Conf. Tetanus*, 1963 (Ed. J.C. Patel); p. 303. Bombay.

Prys-Roberts C., Corbett J.L., Kerr J.H., Smith A.C., Spalding J.M.K. (1969). Treatment of sympathetic overactivity in tetanus. *Lancet*, **1,** 542.

Vakil B.J., Tulpule T.H., Rananvare M.M. (1965). The causes of death in tetanus. *Proc. Int. Conf. Tetanus*, 1963 (Ed. J.C. Patel); p. 282. Bombay.

Wright R. (1960). *The treatment of tetanus.* M.D. Thesis, University of Cape Town.

## CHAPTER 11

Adams E.B. (1968). The prognosis and prevention of tetanus. *S. Afr. med. J.*, **42,** 739.

Adams J.Q., Morton R.F. (1955). Puerperal tetanus. *Amer. J. Obstet. Gynec.*, **69**, 169.

Cole L. (1940). The prognosis of tetanus. *Lancet*, **1**, 164.

Creech O., Glover A., Ochsner A. (1957). Tetanus: Evaluation of treatment at Charity Hospital, New Orleans, Louisiana. *Ann. Surg.*, **146**, 369.

Garcia-Palmieri M.R., Ramirez R. (1957). Generalized tetanus: analysis of 202 cases. *Ann. intern. Med.*, **47**, 721.

Hübner A., Freudenberg K. (1954). Statistique des cas de tetanos en Allemagne. *Rev. Immunol. (Paris)*, **18**, 344.

Huntington R.W., Thompson W.R., Gordon H.H. (1937). The treatment of tetanus with antitoxin. *Ann. Surg.*, **105**, 93.

Johnstone D.D. (1958). Tetanus in Nigeria. Review of 100 cases treated in Ibadan. *Brit. med. J.*, **1**, 12.

Osler W. (1898). *The Principles and Practice of Medicine*, p. 233. Pentland, Edinburgh.

Patel J.C., Joag G.G. (1959). Grading of tetanus to evaluate prognosis. *Indian J. med. Sci.*, **13**, 834.

Patel J.C., Mehta B.C., Modi K.N. (1965*a*). Prognosis in tetanus. *Proc. Int. Conf. Tetanus*, 1963 (Ed. J.C. Patel); p. 181. Bombay.

Patel J.C., Kale P.A., Mehta B.C. (1965*b*). Otogenic tetanus: study of 922 cases. *Ibid.*, p. 158.

Phillips, L.A. (1967). A classification of tetanus. *Lancet*, **1**, 1216.

Sahiar (1944). Some observations on tetanus. *Indian Phycn.*, **3**, 120.

Sanders R.K.M. (1962). *Tetanus in Bihar, India.* M.D. Thesis, University of Bristol.

Tompkins A.B. (1958). Neonatal tetanus in Nigeria. *Brit. med. J.*, **1**, 1382.

Vakil B.J., Aiyer S.N., Tulpule A.T., Mehta A.J., Tulpule T.H. (1965). A study of 2130 cases of tetanus with special reference to incidence, clinical types and prognosis. *Proc. Int. Conf. Tetanus*, 1963 (Ed. J.C. Patel); p. 54. Bombay.

## CHAPTER 12

Armitage P. (1960). *Sequential Medical Trials.* Blackwell, Oxford.

Baker W. de C., Grounds J.G. (1963). Antitetanus serum in the treatment of tetanus. *East Afr. med. J.*, **41**, 93.

Brown A., Mohamed S.D., Montgomery R.D., Armitage P., Laurence D.R. (1960). Value of a large dose of antitoxin in clinical tetanus. *Lancet*, **2**, 227.

Creech O., Glover A., Ochsner A. (1957). Tetanus: Evaluation of treatment at Charity Hospital, New Orleans, Louisiana. *1nn. Surg.*, **146**, 369.

Holloway R. (1966). *Problems in the treatment of tetanus with particular reference to the use of intermittent positive pressure respiration.* M.D. Thesis, University of the Witwatersrand.

Laurence D.R., Webster R.A. (1963). Pathologic physiology, pharmacology and therapeutics of tetanus. *Clin. Pharmacol. Ther.*, **4**, 36.

Lucas A.O., Willis A.J., Mohamed S.D., Montgomery R.D., Steiner H., Armitage P., Laurence D.R. (1965). A comparison of the value of 500,000 I.U. tetanus antitoxin (horse) with 20,000 I.U. in the treatment of tetanus. *Ibid.*, **6**, 592.

Mann N.M., Jackson B.G., Holloway R. (1963). Management of tetanus neonatorum with intermittent positive-pressure respiration. *Arch. Dis. Childh.*, **38**, 251.

Patel J.C., Mehta B.C. (1967). Serum requirements in tetanus. Principles on Tetanus. *Proceedings of an International Conference on Tetanus, Bern,* 1966 (Ed. L. Eckmann); p. 470. Huber, Bern.

Patel J.C., Mehta B.C., Nanavati B.H., Hazra A.K., Rao S.S., Swaminathan C.S. (1963). Role of serum therapy in tetanus. *Lancet*, **1**, 740.

Patel J.C., Rao S.S., Mehta B.C., Goodluck P.L. (1965) Requirement of A.T.S. in non-neonatal tetanus. *Proc. Int. Conf. Tetanus*, 1963 (Ed. J.C. Patel); p. 346. Bombay.

Smith J.W.G. (1967). A comparison of the therapeutic effect of homologous and heterologous tetanus antitoxins. Principles on Tetanus. *Proceedings of an International Conference on Tetanus, Bern,* 1966 (Ed. L. Eckmann); p. 519. Huber, Bern.

Srivastava S.P., Gulati S.P. (1965). Utility of antitetanus serum in treatment of tetanus. *Proc. Int. Conf. Tetanus*, 1963 (Ed. J.C. Patel); p. 363. Bombay.

Tompkins A.B. (1958). Neonatal tetanus in Nigeria. *Brit. med. J.*, **1**, 1382.

Turner T.B., Velasco-Joven E.A., Prudovsky S. (1958). Studies on the prophylaxis and treatment of tetanus II. *Bull. Johns Hopkins Hosp.*, **102**, 71.

Vaishnava H., Passey M.N., Neogy C.N., Gupta S.C., Dixit N.S., Arora N. (1965). Clinical study of tetanus in Delhi for a period of 32 months. *Proc. Int. Conf. Tetanus*, 1963 (Ed. J.C. Patel); p. 33. Bombay.

Vaishnava H., Goyal R.K., Neogy C.N., Mather G.P. (1966). A controlled trial of antiserum in the treatment of tetanus. *Lancet*, **2**, 1371.

Vakil B.J., Tulpule T.H., Armitage P., Laurence D.R. (1963). A comparison of the value of 100,000 I.U. tetanus antitoxin with 50,000 I.U. in the treatment of tetanus. *Clin. Pharmacol. Therap.*, **4**, 182.

Vakil B.J., Tulpule T.H. Armitage P., Laurence D.R. (1964). A comparison of the value of 200,000 I.U. tetanus antitoxin (horse) with 20,000 I.U. in the treatment of tetanus. *Ibid.*, **5**, 695.

Vakil B.J., Tulpule T.H., Armitage P., Laurence D.R. (1968). A comparison of the value of 200,000 I.U. tetanus antitoxin (horse) with 10,000 I.U. in the treatment of tetanus. *Ibid.*, **9**, 465.

Wainwright J.M. (1926). Tetanus, its incidence and treatment. *Arch. Surg.*, **12**, 1062.

Webster R.A., Laurence D.R. (1963). The effect of antitoxin on fixed and free toxin in experimental tetanus. *J. Path. Bact.*, **86**, 413.

Wright G.P. (1955). Neurotoxins of *Clostridium botulinum* and *Clostridium tetani*. *Pharmacol. Rev.*, 7, 413.

## CHAPTER 13

ADAMS E.B. (1958). Clinical Trials in Tetanus. *Proc. roy. Soc. Med.*, **51**, 1002.
ADAMS E.B., WRIGHT R., BERMAN E., LAURENCE D.R. (1959). Treatment of tetanus with chlorpromazine and barbiturates. *Lancet*, **1**, 755.
ADRIANI J., KERR M. (1955). Mephenesin and the combination of mephenesin and chlorpromazine in the management of tetanus. Report of 100 cases. *Sth. med. J. (Bgham, Ala.)*, **48**, 858.
COLE A.C.E., ROBERTSON D.H.H. (1955). Chlorpromazine in the management of tetanus. *Lancet*, **2**, 1063.
CREECH O., GLOVER A., OCHSNER A. (1957). Tetanus: Evaluation of treatment at Charity Hospital, New Orleans, Louisana. *Ann. Surg.*, **146**, 369.
FEMI-PEARSE D. (1966). Experience with diazepam in tetanus. *Brit. med. J.*, **2**, 862.
FORBES G.B., AULD M. (1955). Management of tetanus. Report of fifteen consecutive cases with recovery. *Amer. J. Med.*, **18**, 947.
GELFAND M. (1955). Three cases of tetanus neonatorum successfully treated with chlorpromazine, tetanus antiserum and penicillin. *Cent. Afr. J. Med.*, **1**, 216.
GODMAN H.E., ADRIANI J. (1949). Management of patients with tetanus. *J. Amer. med. Ass.*, **141**, 754.
HARTIGAN J.F. (1884). Trismus nascentium, or the lockjaw of infants. *Amer. J. med. Sci.*, n.s. 87, 84.
HENDRICKSE R.G., SHERMAN P.M. (1966). Tetanus in childhood: Report of a therapeutic trial of diazepam. *Brit. med. J.*, **2**, 860.
ISACSON S.E., SWENSON S.A. (1941). Curare in the treatment of tetanus. *Neb. St. med. J.*, **26**, 136.
KAMAT S.R., PATEL L.R., MUDUR A.N., DHRURA A.J. (1958). Further observations on tetanus. *Curr. med. Pract.*, **2**, 346.
KELLY R.E., LAURENCE D.R. (1956). Effect of chlorpromazine on convulsions of experimental and clinical tetanus. *Lancet*, **1**, 118.
LAURENCE D.R., BERMAN E., SCRAGG J.N., ADAMS E.B. (1958). A clinical trial of chlorpromazine against barbiturates in tetanus. *Ibid.*, **1**, 987.
LAURENCE D.R., WEBSTER R.A. (1961). Tachyphylaxis to the antitetanus activity of some phenothiazines. *Brit. J. Pharmacol.*, **16**, 296.
LAURENCE D.R., WEBSTER R.A. (1963). Pathologic physiology, pharmacology, and therapeutics of tetanus. *Clin. Pharmacol. Ther.*, **4**, 36.
LEWIS R.A., SATOSKAR R.S., JOAG G.C., DAVE B.T., PATEL J.C. (1954). Corticotrophin (ACTH) in severe tetanus. *Indian J. med. Sci.*, **8**, 1.
O'BEIRNE J. (1836). Tetanus, or locked-jaw. *Lancet*, **30**, 826.
PASCALE L.R., WALLYN, R.J., GOLDFEIN S., GUMBINER S.H. (1964). Treatment of tetanus by hyperbaric oxygenation. *J. Amer. med. Ass.*, **189**, 408.
PERLSTEIN M.A., STEIN M.D., ELAM H. (1960). Routine treatment of tetanus. *Ibid.*, **173**, 1536.
POLI E. (1960). The first attempt at curare therapy. *Minerva med.*, **51**, 1411.

RANDALL L.O., HEISE G.A. SCHALLEK W., BAGDON R.E., BANZIGER R., BORIS A., MOE R.A., ABRAMS W.B. (1961). Pharmacological and clinical studies on Valium, a new psychotherapeutic agent of the benzodiazepine class. *Cur. ther. Res.*, **3**, 405.

RHEA J.W., GRAHAM A.W., AKHNOUKH F., PARTHEW C.T. (1967). Effect of hyperbaric oxygenation on neonatal tetanus. *J. Pediat.*, **71**, 33.

RÖ J. (1965). Hyperbaric oxygen treatment following injection of tetanus toxin in mice. *Acta path. microbiol. scand.*, **65**, 421.

SANDERS R.K.M. (1966). Betamethasone in tetanus. *Lancet*, **2**, 1467.

VAN BERGEN F.H., BUCKLEY J.J. (1952). The management of severe systemic tetanus. *Anesthesiology*, **13**, 599.

VERONESI R. (1956). Observations on 712 cases of tetanus subject to four different methods of treatment. *Amer. J. med. Sci.*, **232**, 629.

## CHAPTER 14

*Lancet* (1967). **1**, 886. Tetanus in Britain.

ABLETT J.J.L. (1956). Tetanus and the anaesthetist. *Brit. J. Anaesth.*, **28**, 258.

ADAMS E.B. (1964). Tetanus as a respiratory problem. Results of treatment by means of intermittent positive-pressure respiration. *S. Afr. med. J.*, **38**, 298.

ADAMS E.B., HOLLOWAY R., THAMBIRAN A.K., DESAI S.D. (1966). Usefulness of intermittent positive-pressure respiration in the treatment of tetanus. *Lancet*, **2**, 1176.

BJØRNBOE M., IBSEN B., JOHNSEN S. (1953). Et tilfaelde af tetanus behandlet med curarisering, tracheostomi og overtryksventilation med kvaelstofforilte og ilt. *Ugeskr. Laeg.*, **115**, 1535.

CAMPBELL E.J.M., HOWELL J.B.L. (1960). Simple rapid methods of estimating arterial and mixed venous $Pco^2$. *Brit. med. J.*, **1**, 458.

CLIFTON B. (1964). Hypotension associated with tetanus. *Lancet*, **1**, 785.

COLE L.B., YOUNGMAN H.R., GANDY A.P. (1968). An attack of tetanus. *Ibid.*, **2**, 567.

CREECH O., GLOVER A., OCHSNER A. (1957). Tetanus: Evaluation of treatment at Charity Hospital, New Orleans, Louisiana. *Ann. Surg.*, **146**, 369.

EATON W. L., HOLLOWAY R., SHORT L.J.M. (1967). A multipurpose, modular respiratory monitor for intensive care units using intermittent positive-pressure respiration. *S. Afr. med. J.*, **41**, 499.

GLOSSOP M.W., LOW M.D.W. (1957). Some observations on severe tetanus treated by paralysis and I.P.P.R. *Brit. J. Anaesth.*, **29**, 326.

HERZON E., KILLIAN E., PEARLMAN S.J. (1951). Tracheostomy in tetanus. *Arch. Otolaryng.*, **54**, 143.

HOLLOWAY R. (1967). The place of tracheostomy in tetanus neonatorum. *Arch. Dis. Childh.*, **42**, 546.

HOLLOWAY R., THAMBIRAN A.K. (1967). A self-inflating cuffed neonate tracheostomy tube suitable for intermittent positive-pressure respiration. *Lancet*, **2**, 345.

JACKSON B.G. (1962). *Problems in the technique of intermittent positive-pressure respiration in the treatment of tetanus*. M.D. Thesis, University of London.

MANN N.M., JACKSON B.G., HOLLOWAY R. (1963). Management of tetanus neonatorum with intermittent positive-pressure respiration. *Arch. Dis. Childh.*, **38**, 251.

MOLLARET P., POCIDALO J.J. (1965). Hypoventilation in patients with normal lungs. Management of drug poisoning, tetanus, and myasthenia gravis. *Ann. N.Y. Acad. Sci.*, **121**, 898.

SMITH A.C. (1958). The treatment of severe tetanus by paralysing drugs and intermittent pressure respiration. *Proc. roy. Soc. Med.*, **51**, 1006.

SMYTHE P.M. (1963). Studies on neonatal tetanus and on pulmonary compliance of the totally relaxed infant. *Brit. med. J.*, **1**, 565.

SMYTHE P.M., BULL A. (1959). Treatment of tetanus neonatorum with intermittent positive-pressure respiration. *Ibid.*, **2**, 107.

SYKES M.K. (1960*a*). Observations on a rebreathing technique for the determination of arterial $P_{CO^2}$ in the apnoeic patient. *Brit. J. Anaesth.*, **32**, 256.

SYKES M.K. (1960*b*). Intermittent positive-pressure respiration in tetanus neonatorum. *Anaesthesia*, **15**, 401.

THAMBIRAN A.K. (1967). *Assisted respiration in the treatment of neonatal tetanus*. M.D. Thesis, University of Natal, Durban.

TOREMALM N.G. (1960). A heat and moisture exchanger for post-tracheostomy care. An experimental study. *Acta oto-laryng.* (*Stockh.*), **52**, 461.

WILLIAMS R.E.O., BLOWERS R., GARROD L.P., SHOOTER R.A. (1966). *Hospital infection; causes and prevention*. 2nd Ed. Lloyd Luke, London.

WRIGHT R., SYKES M.K., JACKSON B.G., MANN N.M., ADAMS E.B. (1961). Intermittent positive-pressure respiration in tetanus neonatorum. *Lancet*, **2**, 678.

# INDEX